"The concept of the glycemic index has been distorted and bastardised by popular writers and diet gurus. Here, at last, is a book that explains what we know about the glycemic index and its importance in designing a diet for optimum health. Carbohydrates are not all bad. Read the good news about pasta and even—believe it or not—sugar!"

—ANDREW WEIL, M.D., University of Arizona College of Medicine, author of *Spontaneous Healing* and *8 Weeks to Optimum Health*, on *The New Glucose Revolution*

▼

"Forget *SugarBusters*. Forget *The Zone*. If you want the real scoop on how carbohydrates and sugar affect your body, read this book by the world's leading researchers on the subject. It's the authoritative, last word on choosing foods to control your blood sugar."

—JEAN CARPER, best-selling author of *Miracle Cures, Stop Aging Now!*, and *Food: Your Miracle Medicine*, on *The Glucose Revolution*

▼

"Clear, accessible, and authoritative information about the glycemic index. An exciting, new approach to preventing obesity, diabetes, and heart disease—written by internationally recognized experts in the field."

—DAVID LUDWIG, M.D., PH.D., Director, Obesity Program, Children's Hospital, Boston, on *The New Glucose Revolution*

▼

"Mounting evidence indicates that refined carbohydrates and high glycemic–index foods are contributing to the escalating epidemics of obesity and type 2 diabetes worldwide. This dietary pattern also appears to increase the risk of heart disease and stroke. The skyrocketing proportion of calories from added sugars and refined carbohydrates in Westernized diets portends a future acceleration of these trends. *The Glucose Revolution* challenges traditional doctrines about optimal nutrition and the role of carbohydrates in health and disease. Brand-Miller and colleagues are to be congratulated for an eminently lucid and important book that explains the science behind the glycemic index and provides tools and strategies for modifying diet to incorporate this knowledge. I strongly recommend the book to both health professionals and the general public who could use this state-of-the-art information to improve health and well-being."

—JoAnn E. Manson, M.D., Dr.P.H., Professor of Medicine, Harvard Medical School, and Co-Director of Women's Health, Division of Preventive Medicine, Brigham and Women's Hospital

▼

"Here is at last a book explaining the importance of taking into consideration the glycemic index of foods for overall health, athletic performance, and in reducing the risk of heart disease and diabetes. The book clearly explains that there are different kinds of carbohydrates that work in different ways and why a universal recommendation to "increase the carbohydrate content of your diet" is plainly simple and scientifically inaccurate. Everyone should put the glycemic-index approach into practice."

—Artemis P. Simopoulos, M.D., senior author of
The Omega Diet and *The Healing Diet* and President,
The Center for Genetics, Nutrition and Health,
Washington, D.C., on *The Glucose Revolution*

▼

"*The Glucose Revolution* is nutrition science for the 21st century. Clearly written, it gives the scientific rationale for why all carbohydrates are not created equal. It is a practical guide for both professionals and patients. The food suggestions and recipes are exciting and tasty."

—RICHARD N. PODELL, M.D., M.P.H., Clinical Professor, Department of Family Medicine, UMDNJ-Robert Wood Johnson Medical School, and co-author of *The G-Index Diet: The Missing Link That Makes Permanent Weight Loss Possible*

▼

"Although the jury is still out on the utility of the glycemic index, many of the curious will benefit from a careful reading of this book, and some will find that the glycemic index is particularly helpful for them. Everyone can enjoy the recipes, some of which are to die for!"

—JOHANNA DWYER, D.SC., R.D., editor of *Nutrition Today,* on *The Glucose Revolution*

▼

"The glycemic index is a useful tool which may have a broad spectrum of applications, from the maintenance of fuel supply during exercise to the control of blood glucose levels in diabetics. Low glycemic index foods may prove to have beneficial health effects for all of us in the long term. *The Glucose Revolution* is a user-friendly, easy-to-read overview of all that you need to know about the glycemic index. This book represents a balanced account of the importance of the glycemic index based on sound scientific evidence."

—JAMES HILL, PH.D., Director, Center for Human Nutrition, University of Colorado Health Sciences Center

▼

"*The New Glucose Revolution* summarizes much of the recent development of dietary glycemic index and load in a highly readable format. The authors are able researchers and respected leaders in the nutrition field. Much that is discussed in this book draws directly from their years of experimental and observational research. The focus on dietary intervention and prevention strategies in everyday eating is an especially laudable feature of this book. I recommend this book most highly as an indispensable source of good nutrition."

—SIMIN LIU, M.D., SC.D., Assistant Professor, Department of Epidemiology, Harvard School of Public Health

▼

"As a coach of elite amateur and professional athletes, I know how critical the glycemic index is to sports performance. *The New Glucose Revolution* provides the serious athlete with the basic tools necessary for getting the training table right."

—JOE FRIEL, coach, author, consultant

Other Glucose Revolution Titles

The New Glucose Revolution: The Authoritative Guide to the Glycemic Index—the Dietary Solution for Lifelong Health

The Glucose Revolution Life Plan

■

The Glucose Revolution Pocket Guide to the Top 100 Low Glycemic Foods

The Glucose Revolution Pocket Guide to Diabetes

The Glucose Revolution Pocket Guide to Losing Weight

The Glucose Revolution Pocket Guide to Sports Nutrition

The Glucose Revolution Pocket Guide to Sugar and Energy

The Glucose Revolution Pocket Guide to Your Heart

The Glucose Revolution Pocket Guide to the Glycemic Index and Healthy Kids

The Glucose Revolution Pocket Guide to Children With Type 1 Diabetes

■

FORTHCOMING

The New Glucose Revolution Pocket Guide to Losing Weight

The New Glucose Revolution Pocket Guide to Diabetes

The New Glucose Revolution Pocket Guide to the Metabolic Syndrome and Your Heart

The New Glucose Revolution Pocket Guide to Peak Performance

The New Glucose Revolution Pocket Guide to Healthy Kids

The New Glucose Revolution Pocket Guide to Childhood Diabetes

The NEW GLUCOSE Revolution

COMPLETE GUIDE TO
GLYCEMIC INDEX VALUES

Jennie Brand-Miller, Ph.D.
Johanna Burani, M.S., R.D., C.D.E.
Kaye Foster-Powell, M. Nutr. & Diet.
Susanna Holt, Ph.D

Marlowe & Company
New York

THE NEW GLUCOSE REVOLUTION
COMPLETE GUIDE TO GLYCEMIC INDEX VALUES

Published by
Marlowe & Company
An Imprint of Avalon Publishing Group Incorporated
245 West 17th Street, 11th Floor
New York, NY 10011

This edition published in somewhat different form in Australia in
2003 under the title *The New Glucose Revolution Complete
Guide to GI Values* by Hodder Headline Australia Pty Limited.
This edition is published by arrangement with Hodder Headline
Australia Pty Limited.

Library of Congress Cataloging-in-Publication Data

Brand Miller, Janette, 1952–
The new glucose revolution complete guide to glycemic index values /
by Jennie Brand-Miller, Johanna Burani, Kaye Foster-Powell,
and Susanna Holt.
p. cm.
Includes bibliographical references and index.
ISBN 1-56924-478-2
1. Glycemic index—Handbooks, manuals, etc. 2. Glycemic index—
Tables. I. Title: Pocket guide to the complete glycemic index values.
II. Foster-Powell, Kaye. III. Holt, Susanna. IV. Title.
RC662.B719 2003
613.2'83—dc21   2003052731

9 8 7 6 5 4 3 2

Designed by Pauline Neuwirth, Neuwirth & Associates, Inc.
Printed in the United States of America
Distributed by Publishers Group West

CONTENTS

INTRODUCTION

THE NEW GLUCOSE Revolution Complete Guide to Glycemic Index Values is an essential companion to *The New Glucose Revolution*, the definitive guide to the glycemic index (GI) and its many health benefits. The glycemic index provides you with keys to help you unlock and open the door to better health, increased energy, and lasting weight loss—all through a healthy, satisfying diet.

Although people with certain diet-related conditions, such as diabetes, heart disease, metabolic syndrome (Syndrome X), and excess weight stand to gain the most from acting on our advice, our books offer something for everyone who wants to make wiser food choices, lead a healthier lifestyle, and help to prevent illness in the first place.

This guide will help you put the glycemic index principles into practice. Our book contains three separate Tables:

- an A to Z list of individual foods for easy reference
- a comprehensive list of foods and food categories for more in-depth knowledge
- a simple food-category list in order of GI value low to high, for quick comparisons

You can use the different Tables to:

- find the GI value of your favorite food
- compare foods within the same category (for instance, two types of bread) to see which food has a lower GI value
- improve your diet by finding low-GI substitutes for high-GI foods
- find the lowest GI value within a food group easily
- compare the GI values of food groups
- put together a low-GI meal
- shop for low-GI foods
- check the GI values of products

If you can't find a GI value for a food you eat frequently, look for the closest substitute in the Tables. If there isn't a similar food, the next-best approach is to consider the major ingredient(s) in that food and the manufacturing processes that might affect how quickly the food might be digested into glucose. For example, if you're looking for a GI value for sliced bread, if the flour in that bread is whole grain (not enriched), and is stone-ground (not finely milled by steel blades), its GI value may be similar to a 100 percent stoneground whole-wheat bread.

NOTE: The GI values in this book were correct at press time. The formulation of a commercial food can change, however, which can alter its GI value. For new and revised data, please visit www.glycemicindex.com.

◀ 1 ▶

UNDERSTANDING
THE GLYCEMIC INDEX

*O*UR RESEARCH ON the GI began in the 1980s when health authorities all over the world began to stress the importance of high-carbohydrate diets. Until then, dietary fat had grabbed all the public and scientific attention. (To some extent, this is still true.) But low-fat diets are, by their very nature, automatically high in carbohydrate. That's when we nutrition scientists started asking questions—are all carbohydrates the same, are all starches good for health, are all sugars bad? In particular, we began studying the effects of carbohydrates on blood-glucose levels. We wanted to know which carbohydrate foods were associated with the least fluctuation in blood-glucose levels and with the best overall health, including a reduced risk of diabetes and heart disease.

As we explain in our best-selling book, *The New Glucose Revolution*, the glycemic index:

- is a scientifically proven measure of the effect that carbohydrates have on blood-glucose levels
- helps you choose the right amount and type of carbohydrate for your health and well-being
- provides an easy and effective way to eat a healthy diet and control blood-glucose fluctuations

---

What Is the Glycemic Index?

THE GLYCEMIC INDEX is a physiological measurement of carbohydrate quality—a comparison of carbohydrates, gram for gram, based on their immediate effects on blood-glucose levels.

- Carbohydrates that break down quickly during digestion have high GI values (GI >70). Their blood-glucose response is fast and high.
- Carbohydrates that break down slowly, releasing glucose into the bloodstream gradually, have low GI values (GI <55).

GI Ranges

Low-GI FOODS	55 or less
INTERMEDIATE-GI FOODS	56–69
HIGH-GI FOODS	70 or more

The rate of carbohydrate digestion has important health implications for all of us. For most of us, foods with low GI values have distinct advantages over foods with high GI values, and that's *especially* true if you suffer from diabetes, heart disease, or excess weight.

Once you understand the importance and implications of a food's GI value, you'll be able to choose the right amount and type of carbohydrate to suit your lifestyle. The glycemic index has helped countless people; in fact, it has given many of them a new lease on life!

For more detailed information about the glycemic index, its effects and benefits, you should read our other books, *The New Glucose Revolution* and *The Glucose Revolution Life Plan*. In them, we provide practical advice and tips about changing to a low-GI diet and include lots of delicious recipes, too.

◀ 2 ▶

LET'S TALK GLYCEMIC LOAD

*I*N ADDITION TO the GI values we provide in this book, our Tables also include the glycemic load (GL) value for average-sized food portions. Taken together, the glycemic index and glycemic load values provide you with all the information you need to choose a diet brimming with health-boosting foods.

GLYCEMIC LOAD 101

A food's glycemic load results from the GI value and carbohydrate per serving of food. When we eat a meal containing carbohydrates, our blood-glucose level first rises, then falls. The extent to which it rises and remains high is critically important to our health and depends on two things: The amount of carbohydrate in the meal and the nature (GI value) of that carbohydrate. Both factors equally determine blood-glucose changes.

Researchers at Harvard University came up with a way of combining and describing these two factors with the term "glycemic load," which not only provides a measure of the level of glucose in the blood, but also the insulin demand produced by a normal serving of the food. Researchers measure GI values for fixed portions of foods containing a certain amount of carbohydrate (usually 50 grams). Then, as people eat different-sized portions of the same foods, we can work out the extent to which a certain portion of food will raise the blood-glucose level by calculating a glycemic load value for that amount of food.

To calculate glycemic load, multiply a food's GI value by the amount of carbohydrate in a particular serving size, then divide by 100.

■

Glycemic load = (GI x carbohydrate per serving) ÷ 100

■

For example, a small apple has a GI value of 40 and contains 15 grams of carbohydrate. Its glycemic load is $(40 \times 15) \div 100 = 6$. A small 5-ounce potato has a GI value of 90 and 15 grams of carbohydrate. It has a glycemic load of $(90 \times 15) \div 100 = 14$. This means one small potato will raise your blood-glucose level higher than one apple.

How GI Values Affect Glycemic Load

THE GLYCEMIC LOAD is greatest for those foods that provide the highest-GI carbohydrate, particularly those we tend to eat in large quantities. Compare the glycemic load of the following foods to see how the serving size, as well as the GI value, help to determine the glycemic response:

Rice, 1 cup
Carbohydrates: 43
GI: 83
GL: 36
(83 × 43) ÷ 100 = 36

Spaghetti, 1 cup
Carbohydrates: 40
GI: 44
GL: 18
(44 × 40) ÷ 100 = 18

Some nutritionists argue that the glycemic load is an improvement on the glycemic index because it provides an estimate of both quantity and quality of carbohydrate (the GI just gives us quality) in a diet. In large Harvard studies, however, researchers were able to predict disease risk from people's overall diet, as well as its glycemic load. Using the glycemic load strengthened the relationship, suggesting that the more frequently we consume high carbohydrate, high-GI foods, the worse it is for our health. Carbohydrate by itself has no effect; in other words, there was no benefit to low carbohydrate intake over high carbohydrate intake, or vice versa.

■
Low GL = 10 or less
Intermediate GL = 11–19
High GL = 20 or more
■

If you make the mistake of using GL alone, you might find yourself eating a diet with very little carbohydrate but a lot of fat and excessive amounts of protein. That's why you need to use the GI to compare foods of similar nature (such as bread with bread) and use the glycemic load when you're deciding on the portion size of the carbohydrates you want to eat. If you use the technique correctly, GL values will guide you to eat smaller portions of high GI foods.

Remember that the GL values we provide are for the nominal, or standardized, portion sizes listed. If you eat a different portion size, then you'll need to calculate another GI value. Here's how: First, determine the size of your portion, then work out the available carbohydrate content of this weight (this value is listed next to the GL), then multiply by the food's GI value. For example, the nominal serving size listed for bran flakes is $\frac{1}{2}$ cup, the available carbohydrate is 18 grams, and the GI is 74. So the GL for a $\frac{1}{2}$-cup serving of bran flakes is $(74 \times 18) \div 100 = 13$. If, however, you normally eat 1 cup of bran flakes, you'd need to double the available carbohydrate $(18 \times 2 = 36)$ and the GL for your larger cereal portion would be $(74 \times 36) \div 100 = 27$. These numbers show that the larger portion of cereal releases a larger quantity of glucose into the bloodstream.

◀ 3 ▶

YOUR DAILY FOOD CHOICES

To HELP GUIDE your daily food choices, we've created two GI Food Pyramids, one for moderate carbohydrate eaters and one for high carbohydrate eaters. The recommended servings of each food group are shown on each pyramid. If you are a big bread and cereal eater, the GI Food Pyramid for high carbohydrate eaters will suit you best. Either way, the serving information on pages 12–13 applies to both pyramids.

Changes on the Way

MEDICAL AND SCIENTIFIC researchers are now scrutinizing the current structure of the USDA Food Guide Pyramid and are likely to recommend some changes in the near future. That's why the serving sizes we suggest in the following two Glycemic Index Food Pyramids reflect the guidelines established by the Institute of Nutrition of the American Academy of Science.

The Glycemic Index Food Pyramid
For MODERATE Carbohydrate Eaters

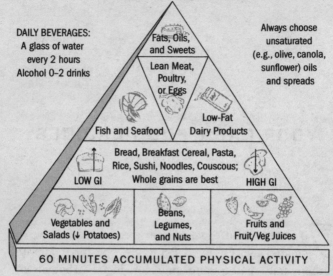

DAILY BEVERAGES:
A glass of water
every 2 hours
Alcohol 0–2 drinks

Always choose
unsaturated
(e.g., olive, canola,
sunflower) oils
and spreads

Fats, Oils,
and Sweets

Lean Meat,
Poultry,
or Eggs

Fish and Seafood

Low-Fat
Dairy Products

Bread, Breakfast Cereal, Pasta,
Rice, Sushi, Noodles, Couscous;
Whole grains are best

LOW GI

HIGH GI

Vegetables and
Salads (↓ Potatoes)

Beans,
Legumes,
and Nuts

Fruits and
Fruit/Veg Juices

60 MINUTES ACCUMULATED PHYSICAL ACTIVITY

DAILY

For moderate carbohydrate eaters:

Fats, oils, and sweets: 1–2 servings

Fish, seafood, lean meat, poultry, and eggs:
3–4 servings

Low-fat dairy products: 3–4 servings

Bread, breakfast cereals, and grains: 4–6 servings

Vegetables and salads: 4–6 servings

Beans, legumes, and nuts: 1–2 servings

Fruits and juices: 2–3 servings

The Glycemic Index Food Pyramid
For HIGH Carbohydrate Eaters

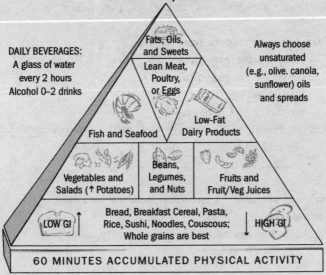

DAILY BEVERAGES:
A glass of water
every 2 hours
Alcohol 0–2 drinks

Always choose
unsaturated
(e.g., olive, canola,
sunflower) oils
and spreads

Fats, Oils,
and Sweets

Lean Meat,
Poultry,
or Eggs

Fish and Seafood

Low-Fat
Dairy Products

Vegetables and
Salads (↑ Potatoes)

Beans,
Legumes,
and Nuts

Fruits and
Fruit/Veg Juices

LOW GI ↑

Bread, Breakfast Cereal, Pasta,
Rice, Sushi, Noodles, Couscous;
Whole grains are best

↓ HIGH GI

60 MINUTES ACCUMULATED PHYSICAL ACTIVITY

DAILY

For high carbohydrate eaters:

Fats, oils, and sweets: 1–2 servings

Fish, seafood, lean meat, poultry, and eggs:
2–3 servings

Low-fat dairy products: 2–3 servings

Bread, breakfast cereals, and grains: 6–8 servings

Vegetables and salads: 4–6 servings

Beans, legumes, and nuts: 1 serving

Fruits and juices: 3–4 servings

SERVING INFORMATION

These serving sizes apply to both GI Pyramids.

Fats, oils, and sweets (one serving):
   1 Tbsp butter, margarine, oil
   2 Tbsp cream, mayonnaise
   1 oz chocolate
   1 small slice (1½ oz) cake
   ¾ oz (about 9–13 chips) snack pack potato chips
   1 standard alcoholic drink (1.5 oz); wine (5 oz);
      beer (12 oz)

Fish and seafood / Lean meat, poultry, and eggs (one serving):
   2½ to 3 oz cooked lean meat, poultry, or fish
   1 egg = 1 oz meat

Low-fat dairy products (one serving):
   1 cup low-fat milk or yogurt
   1½ to 2 oz reduced-fat cheese
   1½ cups iced milk
   1 cup frozen yogurt

Bread, breakfast cereals, grains, etc. (one serving):
   1 slice bread
   1 oz cereal, ready-to-eat
   ½ cup cooked cereal, rice, pasta, or noodles

Vegetables and salads (one serving):

   ½ cup cooked vegetables

   1 cup raw, leafy vegetables

Beans, legumes, and nuts (one serving):

   1 cup cooked dried beans, peas, or lentils

   ⅓ cup nuts = 1 oz meat

   2 Tbsp peanut butter = 1 oz meat

Fruits and juices (one serving):

   1 medium piece of fruit

   ½ cup of sliced, cooked, or canned fruit

   ¾ cup fruit juice

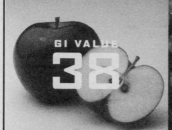

GI VALUE
38

GI VALUE
53

GI VALUE
29

GI VALUE
38

GI VALUE
59

GI VALUE
42

GI VALUE
46

GI VALUE
44

THE TABLES

KEY TO THE TABLES

GI: The glycemic index for the food, where glucose equals 100

NOMINAL SERVING SIZE: The portion of food tested

NET CARB PER SERVING: The total grams of carbs available to the body for digestion from the particular food in the specific serving size (total grams of carbs minus grams of fiber)

GL PER SERVING: Glycemic load of the food; this relates to the quantity of carbs that will enter the bloodstream for the particular food in the specific serving size

◀ 4 ▶

A TO Z GI VALUES

THE TABLES IN this section will help you find a food's glycemic index value quickly and easily, because we've listed the foods alphabetically.

The list provides not only the food's glycemic index value but also its glycemic load [GL = (carbohydrate content × GI) ÷ 100]. We calculate the glycemic load using a nominal serving size as well as the carbohydrate content of that serving—both of which we've also listed. That way, you can choose foods with either a low GI value or a low glycemic load. If your favorite food is both high GI and high GL, you can either cut down the serving size or dilute the GL by combining it with very low-GI foods—for example, eating rice (high GI) with lentils (low GI).

For the first time, we've also included foods that have very little carbohydrate; their GI value is zero, indicated by [0]. Many vegetables, such as avocados and broccoli, and protein foods such as chicken, cheese, and tuna, fall into the low- or no-carbohydrate category. Most alcoholic beverages are also low in carbohydrate.

FOOD	GI Value	Nominal Serving Size	Net Carb per Serving	GI per Serving
A				
All-Bran®, breakfast cereal	30	½ cup	15	4
Almonds	[0]	1.75 oz	0	0
Angel food cake, 1 slice	67	¹⁄₁₂ cake	29	19
Apple, dried	29	9 rings	34	10
Apple, fresh, medium	38	4 oz	15	6
Apple juice, pure, unsweetened, reconstituted	40	8 oz	29	12
Apple muffin, small	44	3.5 oz	41	18
Apricots, canned in light syrup	64	4 halves	19	12
Apricots, dried	30	17 halves	27	8
Apricots, fresh, 3 medium	57	4 oz	9	5
Arborio, risotto rice, cooked	69	¾ cup	53	36
Artichokes (Jerusalem)	[0]	½ cup	0	0
Avocado	[0]	¼	0	0
B				
Bagel, white	72	½	35	25
Baked beans	38	⅔ cup	31	12
Baked beans, canned in tomato sauce	48	⅔ cup	15	7
Banana cake, 1 slice	47	⅛ cake	38	18
Banana, fresh, medium	52	4 oz	24	12
Barley, pearled, cooked	25	1 cup	42	11
Basmati rice, white, cooked	58	1 cup	38	22
Beef	[0]	4 oz	0	0
Beer	[0]	8 oz	10	0
Beets, canned	64	½ cup	7	5
Bengal gram dhal, chickpea	11	5 oz	36	4
Black bean soup	64	1 cup	27	17
Black beans, cooked	30	⅘ cup	23	7
Black-eyed peas, canned	42	⅔ cup	17	7

[0] indicates that the food has so little carbohydrate that the GI value cannot be tested. The GL, therefore, is 0.

FOOD	GI Value	Nominal Serving Size	Net Carb per Serving	GL per Serving
Blueberry muffin, small	59	3.5 oz	47	28
Bok choy, raw	[0]	1 cup	0	0
Bran Flakes™, breakfast cereal	74	½ cup	18	13
Bran muffin, small	60	3.5 oz	41	25
Brandy	[0]	1 oz	0	0
Brazil nuts	[0]	1.75 oz	0	0
Breton wheat crackers	67	6 crackers	14	10
Broad beans	79	½ cup	11	9
Broccoli, raw	[0]	1 cup	0	0
Broken rice, white, cooked	86	1 cup	43	37
Brown rice, cooked	50	1 cup	33	16
Buckwheat	54	¾ cup	30	16
Bulgur, cooked 20 min	48	¾ cup	26	12
Bun, hamburger	61	1.5 oz	22	13
Butter beans, canned	31	⅔ cup	20	6

C

FOOD	GI Value	Nominal Serving Size	Net Carb per Serving	GL per Serving
Cabbage, raw	[0]	1 cup	0	0
Cactus Nectar, Organic Agave, light, 90% fructose (Western Commerce)	11	1 Tbsp	8	1
Cactus Nectar, Organic Agave, light, 97% fructose (Western Commerce)	10	1 Tbsp	8	1
Cantaloupe, fresh	65	4 oz	6	4
Capellini pasta, cooked	45	1½ cups	45	20
Carrot juice, fresh	43	8 oz	23	10
Carrots, peeled, cooked	49	½ cup	5	2
Carrots, raw	47	1 medium	6	3
Cashew nuts, salted	22	1.75 oz	13	3
Cauliflower, raw	[0]	¾ cup	0	0
Celery, raw	[0]	2 stalks	0	0
Cheese	[0]	4 oz	0	0

[0] indicates that the food has so little carbohydrate that the GI value cannot be tested. The GL, therefore, is 0.

FOOD	GI Value	Nominal Serving Size	Net Carb per Serving	GL per Serving
Cherries, fresh	22	18	12	3
Chicken nuggets, frozen	46	4 oz	16	7
Chickpeas, canned	42	⅔ cup	22	9
Chickpeas, dried, cooked	28	⅔ cup	30	8
Chocolate cake made from mix with chocolate frosting	38	4 oz	52	20
Chocolate milk, low-fat	34	8 oz	26	9
Chocolate mousse, 2% fat	31	½ cup	22	7
Chocolate powder, dissolved in water	55	8 oz	16	9
Chocolate pudding, made from powder and whole milk	47	½ cup	24	11
Choice DM™, nutritional support product, vanilla (Mead Johnson)	23	8 oz	24	6
Clif® bar (cookies & cream)	101	2.4 oz	34	34
Coca Cola®, soft drink	53	8 oz	26	14
Cocoa Puffs™, breakfast cereal	77	1 cup	26	20
Complete™, breakfast cereal	48	1 cup	21	10
Condensed milk, sweetened	61	2½ Tbsps	27	17
Converted rice, long-grain, cooked 20-30 min, Uncle Ben's	50	1 cup	36	18
Converted rice, white, cooked 20-30 min, Uncle Ben's	38	1 cup	36	14
Corn Flakes™, breakfast cereal	92	1 cup	26	24
Corn Flakes™, Honey Crunch, breakfast cereal	72	¾ cup	25	18
Corn pasta, gluten-free	78	1¼ cups	42	32
Corn Pops™, breakfast cereal	80	1 cup	26	21
Corn Thins, puffed corn cakes, gluten-free	87	1 oz	20	18
Corn, sweet, cooked	60	½ cup	18	11
Cornmeal, cooked 2 min	68	1 cup	13	9
Couscous, cooked 5 min	65	¾ cup	35	23

[0] indicates that the food has so little carbohydrate that the GI value cannot be tested. The GL, therefore, is 0.

FOOD	GI Value	Nominal Serving Size	Net Carb per Serving	GL per Serving
Cranberry juice cocktail	52	8 oz	31	16
Crispix™, breakfast cereal	87	1 cup	25	22
Croissant, medium	67	2 oz	26	17
Cucumber, raw	[0]	¾ cup	0	0
Cupcake, strawberry-iced, small	73	1.5 oz	26	19
Custard apple, raw, flesh only	54	4 oz	19	10
Custard, homemade	43	½ cup	26	11
Custard, prepared from powder with whole milk, instant	35	½ cup	26	9

D

FOOD	GI Value	Nominal Serving Size	Net Carb per Serving	GL per Serving
Dates, dried	50	7	40	20
Desiree potato, peeled, cooked	101	5 oz	17	17
Doughnut, cake type	76	1.75 oz	23	17

E

FOOD	GI Value	Nominal Serving Size	Net Carb per Serving	GL per Serving
Eggs, large	[0]	2	0	0
Enercal Plus™ (Wyeth-Ayerst)	61	8 oz	40	24
English Muffin™ bread (Natural Ovens)	77	1 oz	14	11
Ensure™, vanilla drink	48	8 oz	34	16
Ensure™ bar, chocolate fudge brownie	43	1.4 oz	20	8
Ensure Plus™, vanilla drink	40	8 oz	47	19
Ensure Pudding™, old-fashioned vanilla	36	4 oz	26	9

F

FOOD	GI Value	Nominal Serving Size	Net Carb per Serving	GL per Serving
Fanta®, orange soft drink	68	8 oz	34	23
Fettuccine, egg, cooked	32	1½ cups	46	15
Figs, dried	61	3	26	16
Fish	[0]	4 oz	0	0
Fish sticks	38	3.5 oz	19	7
Flan/crème caramel	65	½ cup	73	47
French baguette, white, plain	95	1 oz	15	15

[0] indicates that the food has so little carbohydrate that the GI value cannot be tested. The GL, therefore, is 0.

FOOD	QI Value	Nominal Serving Size	Net Carb per Serving	GL per Serving
French fries, frozen, reheated in microwave	75	30 pcs	29	22
French green beans, cooked	[0]	½ cup	0	0
French vanilla cake made from mix, with vanilla frosting	42	4 oz	58	24
French vanilla ice cream, premium, 16% fat	38	½ cup	14	5
Froot Loops™, breakfast cereal	69	1 cup	26	18
Frosted Flakes™, breakfast cereal	55	1 cup	26	15
Fructose, pure	19	1 Tbsp	10	2
Fruit cocktail, canned, light syrup	55	½ cup	16	9
Fruit leather	61	2 pcs	24	15
G				
Gatorade™ (orange) sports drink	89	8 oz	15	13
Gin	[0]	1 oz	0	0
Glucerna™, vanilla (Abbott)	31	8 oz	23	7
Glucose (dextrose)	99	1 Tbsp	10	10
Glucose tablets	102	3 pcs	15	15
Gluten-free corn pasta	78	1½ cups	42	32
Gluten-free multigrain bread	79	1 oz	13	10
Gluten-free rice and corn pasta	76	1½ cups	49	37
Gluten-free spaghetti, rice and split pea, canned in tomato sauce	68	8 oz	27	19
Gluten-free split pea and soy pasta shells	29	1½ cups	31	9
Gluten-free white bread, sliced	80	1 oz	15	12
Glutinous (sticky) rice, white, cooked	92	⅔ cup	48	44
Gnocchi	68	6 oz	48	33
Grapefruit juice, unsweetened	48	8 oz	20	9
Grapefruit, fresh, medium	25	1 half	11	3
Grape-Nuts® (Post), breakfast cereal	75	¼ cup	21	16

[0] indicates that the food has so little carbohydrate that the GI value cannot be tested. The GL, therefore, is 0.

FOOD	GI Value	Nominal Serving Size	Net Carb per Serving	GL per Serving
Grapes, black, fresh	59	¾ cup	18	11
Grapes, green, fresh	46	¾ cup	18	8
Green peas	48	⅓ cup	7	3
Green pea soup, canned	66	8 oz	41	27
H				
Hamburger bun	61	1.5 oz	22	13
Happiness™ (cinnamon, raisin, pecan bread) (Natural Ovens)	63	1 oz	14	9
Hazelnuts	[0]	1.75 oz	0	0
Healthy Choice™ Hearty 100% Whole Grain	62	1 oz	14	9
Healthy Choice™ Hearty 7-Grain	55	1 oz	14	8
Honey	55	1 Tbsp	18	10
Hot cereal, apple & cinnamon, dry (Con Agra)	37	1.2 oz	22	8
Hot cereal, unflavored, dry (Con Agra)	25	1.2 oz	19	5
Hunger Filler™, whole-grain bread (Natural Ovens)	59	1 oz	13	7
I				
Ice cream, low-fat, vanilla, "light"	50	½ cup	9	5
Ice cream, premium, French vanilla, 16% fat	38	½ cup	14	5
Ice cream, premium, "ultra chocolate," 15% fat	37	½ cup	14	5
Ice cream, regular fat	61	½ cup	20	12
Instant potato, mashed	97	¾ cup	20	17
Instant rice, white, cooked 6 min	87	¾ cup	42	36
Ironman PR® bar, chocolate	39	2.3 oz	26	10

[0] indicates that the food has so little carbohydrate that the GI value cannot be tested. The GL, therefore, is 0.

FOOD	GI Value	Nominal Serving Size	Net Carb per Serving	GL per Serving
J				
Jam, apricot fruit spread, reduced sugar	55	1½ Tbsps	13	7
Jam, strawberry	51	1½ Tbsps	20	10
Jasmine rice, white, cooked	109	1 cup	42	46
Jelly beans	78	10 large	28	22
K				
Kaiser roll	73	1 half	16	12
Kavli™ Norwegian crispbread	71	5 pcs	16	12
Kidney beans, canned	52	⅔ cup	17	9
Kidney beans, cooked	23	⅔ cup	25	6
Kiwi fruit	53	4 oz	12	7
Kudos® Whole Grain Bars, chocolate chip	62	1.8 oz	32	20
L				
Lactose, pure	46	1 Tbsp	10	5
Lamb	[0]	4 oz	0	0
Leafy vegetables (spinach, arugula, etc.), raw	[0]	1½ cups	0	0
L.E.A.N Fibergy™ bar, Harvest Oat	45	1.75 oz	29	13
L.E.A.N Life long Nutribar™, Chocolate Crunch	32	1.5 oz	19	6
L.E.A.N Life long Nutribar™, Peanut Crunch	30	1.5 oz	19	6
L.E.A.N Nutrimeal™, drink powder, Dutch Chocolate	26	8 oz	13	3
Lemonade, reconstituted	66	8 oz	20	13
Lentil soup, canned	44	9 oz	21	9
Lentils, brown, cooked	29	¾ cup	18	5
Lentils, green, cooked	30	¾ cup	17	5
Lentils, red, cooked	26	¾ cup	18	5

[0] indicates that the food has so little carbohydrate that the GI value cannot be tested. The GL, therefore, is 0.

FOOD	GI Value	Nominal Serving Size	Net Carb per Serving	GL per Serving
Lettuce	[0]	4 leaves	0	0
Life Savers®, peppermint candy	70	18 pcs	30	21
Light rye bread	68	1 oz	14	10
Lima beans, baby, frozen	32	¾ cup	30	10
Linguine pasta, thick, cooked	46	1½ cups	48	22
Linguine pasta, thin, cooked	52	1½ cups	45	23
Long-grain rice, cooked 10 min	61	1 cup	36	22
Lychees, canned in syrup, drained	79	4 oz	20	16

M

FOOD	GI Value	Nominal Serving Size	Net Carb per Serving	GL per Serving
M & M's®, peanut	33	15 pcs	17	6
Macadamia nuts	[0]	1.75 oz	0	0
Macaroni and cheese, made from mix	64	1 cup	51	32
Macaroni, cooked	47	1¼ cups	48	23
Maltose	105	1 Tbsp	10	11
Mango	51	4 oz	15	8
Maple syrup, pure Canadian	54	1 Tbsp	18	10
Marmalade, orange	48	1½ Tbsps	20	9
Mars Bar®	68	2 oz	40	27
Melba toast, Old London	70	6 pcs	23	16
METRx® bar (vanilla)	74	3.6 oz	50	37
Milk Arrowroot™ cookies	69	5	18	12
Millet, cooked	71	⅔ cup	36	25
Mini Wheats™, whole-wheat breakfast cereal	58	12 pcs	21	12
Mousse, butterscotch, 1.9% fat	36	1.75 oz	10	4
Mousse, chocolate, 2% fat	31	1.75 oz	11	3
Mousse, hazelnut, 2.4% fat	36	1.75 oz	10	4
Mousse, mango, 1.8% fat	33	1.75 oz	11	4
Mousse, mixed berry, 2.2% fat	36	1.75 oz	10	4
Mousse, strawberry, 2.3% fat	32	1.75 oz	10	3

[0] indicates that the food has so little carbohydrate that the GI value cannot be tested. The GL, therefore, is 0.

FOOD	GI Value	Nominal Serving Size	Net Carb per Serving	GL per Serving
Muesli bar containing dried fruit	61	1 oz	21	13
Muesli bread, made from mix in bread oven (Con Agra)	54	1 oz	12	7
Muesli, gluten-free, with low-fat milk	39	1 oz	19	7
Muesli, Swiss Formula	56	1 oz	16	9
Muesli, toasted	43	1 oz	17	7
Multi-Grain 9-Grain bread	43	1 oz	14	6
N				
Navy beans, canned	38	5 oz	31	12
Nesquik™, chocolate dissolved in low-fat milk, no-sugar-added	41	8 oz	11	5
Nesquik™, strawberry dissolved in low-fat milk, no-sugar-added	35	8 oz	12	4
New creamer potato, canned	65	5 oz	18	12
New creamer potato, unpeeled and cooked 20 min	78	5 oz	21	16
Noodles, instant "two-minute" (Maggi®)	46	1½ cups	40	19
Noodles, mung bean (Lungkow beanthread), dried, cooked	39	1½ cups	45	18
Noodles, rice, fresh, cooked	40	1½ cups	39	15
Nutella®, chocolate hazelnut spread	33	1 Tbsp	12	4
Nutrigrain™, breakfast cereal	66	1 cup	15	10
Nutty Natural™, whole-grain bread (Natural Ovens)	59	1 oz	12	7
O				
Oat bran, raw	55	2 Tbsp	5	3
Oatmeal, cooked 1 min	66	1 cup	26	17
Oatmeal cookies	55	4 small	21	12
Orange juice, unsweetened, reconstituted	53	8 oz	18	9
Orange, fresh, medium	42	4 oz	11	5

[0] indicates that the food has so little carbohydrate that the GI value cannot be tested. The GL, therefore, is 0.

FOOD	GI Value	Nominal Serving Size	Net Carb per Serving	GL per Serving
P				
Pancakes, buckwheat, gluten-free, made from mix	102	2 4″ pancakes	22	22
Pancakes, made from mix	67	2 4″ pancakes	58	39
Papaya, fresh	59	4 oz	8	5
Parsnips	97	½ cup	12	12
Pastry	59	2 oz	26	15
Pea soup, canned	66	8 oz	41	27
Peach, canned in heavy syrup	58	½ cup	26	15
Peach, canned in light syrup	52	½ cup	18	9
Peach, fresh, large	42	4 oz	11	5
Peanuts	14	1.75 oz	6	1
Pear halves, canned in natural juice	43	½ cup	13	5
Pear, fresh	38	4 oz	11	4
Peas, green, frozen, cooked	48	½ cup	7	3
Pecans	[0]	1.75 oz	0	0
Pepper, fresh, green or red	[0]	3 oz	0	0
Pineapple juice, unsweetened	46	8 oz	34	15
Pineapple, fresh	66	4 oz	10	6
Pinto beans, canned	45	⅔ cup	22	10
Pinto beans, dried, cooked	39	¾ cup	26	10
Pita bread, white	57	1 oz	17	10
Pizza, cheese	60	1 slice	27	16
Pizza, Super Supreme, pan (11.4% fat)	36	1 slice	24	9
Pizza, Super Supreme, thin and crispy (13.2% fat)	30	1 slice	22	7
Plums, fresh	39	2 medium	12	5
Pop Tarts™, double chocolate	70	1.8 oz pastry	36	25
Popcorn, plain, cooked in microwave oven	72	1½ cups	11	8
Pork	[0]	4 oz	0	0

[0] indicates that the food has so little carbohydrate that the GI value cannot be tested. The GL, therefore, is 0.

FOOD	GI Value	Nominal Serving Size	Net Carb per Serving	GL per Serving
Potato chips, plain, salted	54	2 oz	21	11
Potato, baked	85	5 oz	30	26
Potato, microwaved	82	5 oz	33	27
Pound cake (Sara Lee)	54	2 oz	28	15
PowerBar® (chocolate)	57	2.3 oz	42	24
Premium soda crackers	74	5 crackers	17	12
Pretzels	83	1 oz	20	16
Prunes, pitted	29	6	33	10
Pudding, instant, chocolate, made with whole milk	47	½ cup	24	11
Pudding, instant, vanilla, made with whole milk	40	½ cup	24	10
Puffed crispbread	81	1 oz	19	15
Puffed rice cakes, white	82	3 cakes	21	17
Puffed Wheat, breakfast cereal	80	2 cups	21	17
Pumpernickel rye kernel bread	41	1 oz	12	5
Pumpkin	75	3 oz	4	3
R				
Raisin Bran™, breakfast cereal	61	½ cup	19	12
Raisins	64	½ cup	44	28
Ravioli, meat-filled, cooked	39	6.5 oz	38	15
Red wine	[0]	3.5 oz	0	0
Red-skinned potato, peeled and microwaved on high for 6–7.5 min	79	5 oz	18	14
Red-skinned potato, peeled, boiled 35 min	88	5 oz	18	16
Red-skinned potato, peeled, mashed	91	5 oz	20	18
Resource Diabetic™, nutritional support product, vanilla (Novartis)	34	8 oz	23	8
Rice and corn pasta, gluten-free	76	1½ cups	49	37
Rice bran, extruded	19	1 oz	14	3

[0] indicates that the food has so little carbohydrate that the GI value cannot be tested. The GL, therefore, is 0.

FOOD	GI Value	Nominal Serving Size	Net Carb per Serving	GL per Serving
Rice cakes, white	82	3 cakes	21	17
Rice Krispies Treat™ bar	63	1 oz	24	15
Rice Krispies™, breakfast cereal	82	1¼ cups	26	22
Rice noodles, fresh, cooked	40	1½ cups	39	15
Rice, parboiled	72	1 cup	36	26
Rice pasta, brown, cooked 16 min	92	1½ cups	38	35
Rice vermicelli	58	1½ cups	39	22
Rolled oats	42	1 cup	21	9
Roll-Ups®, processed fruit snack	99	1 oz	25	24
Roman (cranberry) beans, fresh, cooked	46	¾ cup	18	8
Russet, baked potato	85	5 oz	30	26
Rutabaga, fresh, cooked	72	5 oz	10	7
Rye bread	58	1 oz	14	8
Ryvita® crackers	69	3 crackers	16	11
S				
Salami	[0]	4 oz	0	0
Salmon	[0]	4 oz	0	0
Sausages, fried	28	3.5 oz	3	1
Scones, plain	92	1 oz	9	8
Sebago potato, peeled, cooked	87	5 oz	17	14
Seeded rye bread	55	1 oz	13	7
Semolina, cooked (dry)	55	⅓ cup	50	28
Shellfish (shrimp, crab, lobster, etc.)	[0]	4 oz	0	0
Sherry	[0]	2 oz	0	0
Shortbread cookies	64	1 oz	16	10
Shredded Wheat™, breakfast cereal	75	⅔ cup	20	15
Shredded Wheat™ biscuits	62	1 oz	18	11
Skim milk	32	8 oz	13	4
Skittles®	70	45 pcs	45	32

[0] indicates that the food has so little carbohydrate that the GI value cannot be tested. The GL, therefore, is 0.

FOOD	GI Value	Nominal Serving Size	Net Carb per Serving	GL per Serving
Smacks™, breakfast cereal	71	¾ cup	23	11
Smoothie, raspberry (Con Agra)	33	8 oz	41	14
Snack bar, Apple Cinnamon (Con Agra)	40	1.75 oz	29	12
Snack bar, Peanut Butter & Choc-Chip (Con Agra)	37	1.75 oz	27	10
Snickers® bar	68	2.2 oz	35	23
Soda Crackers, Premium	74	5 crackers	17	12
Soft drink, Coca Cola®	53	8 oz	26	14
Soft drink, Fanta®, orange	68	8 oz	34	23
Sourdough rye	48	1 oz	12	6
Sourdough wheat	54	1 oz	14	8
Soy & Flaxseed bread (mix in bread oven) (Con Agra)	50	1 oz	10	5
Soybeans, canned	14	1 cup	6	1
Soybeans, dried, cooked	20	1 cup	6	1
Spaghetti, durum wheat, cooked 20 min	64	1½ cups	43	27
Spaghetti, gluten-free, rice and split pea, canned in tomato sauce	68	8 oz	27	19
Spaghetti, white, cooked 5 min	38	1½ cups	48	18
Spaghetti, whole wheat, cooked 5 min	32	1½ cups	44	14
Special K™, breakfast cereal	69	1 cup	21	14
Spirali pasta, durum wheat, al dente	43	1½ cups	44	19
Split pea and soy pasta shells, gluten-free	29	1½ cups	31	9
Split-pea soup	60	1 cup	27	16
Split peas, yellow, cooked 20 min	32	¾ cup	19	6
Sponge cake, plain	46	2 oz	36	17
Squash, raw	[0]	⅔ cup	0	0
Star pastina, white, cooked 5 min	38	1½ cups	48	18

[0] indicates that the food has so little carbohydrate that the GI value cannot be tested. The GL, therefore, is 0.

FOOD	GI Value	Nominal Serving Size	Net Carb per Serving	GL per Serving
Stay Trim™, whole-grain bread (Natural Ovens)	70	1 oz	15	10
Stoned Wheat Thins	67	14 crackers	17	12
Strawberries, fresh	40	4 oz	3	1
Strawberry jam	51	1½ Tbsps	20	10
Strawberry shortcake	42	2.2 oz	40	17
Stuffing, bread	74	1 oz	21	16
Sucrose	68	1 Tbsp	10	7
Super Supreme pizza, pan (11.4% fat)	36	1 slice	24	9
Super Supreme pizza, thin and crispy (13.2% fat)	30	1 slice	22	7
Sushi, salmon	48	3.5 oz	36	17
Sweet corn, whole kernel, canned, diet-pack, drained	46	1 cup	28	13
Sweet potato, cooked	44	5 oz	25	11

T

FOOD	GI Value	Nominal Serving Size	Net Carb per Serving	GL per Serving
Taco shells, baked	68	2 shells	12	8
Tapioca, cooked with milk	81	¾ cup	18	14
Tofu-based frozen dessert, chocolate with high-fructose (24%) corn syrup	115	1.75 oz	9	10
Tomato juice, canned, no added sugar	38	8 oz	9	4
Tomato soup	38	1 cup	17	6
Tortellini, cheese	50	6.5 oz	21	10
Tortilla chips, plain, salted	63	1.75 oz	26	17
Total™, breakfast cereal	76	¾ cup	22	17
Tuna	[0]	4 oz	0	0
Twix® Cookie Bar, caramel	44	2 cookies	39	17

U

FOOD	GI Value	Nominal Serving Size	Net Carb per Serving	GL per Serving
Ultra chocolate ice cream, premium, 15% fat	37	½ cup	14	5
Ultracal™ with fiber (Mead Johnson)	40	8 oz	29	12

[0] indicates that the food has so little carbohydrate that the GI value cannot be tested. The GL, therefore, is 0.

FOOD	GI Value	Nominal Serving Size	Net Carb per Serving	GL per Serving
V				
Vanilla cake made from mix, with vanilla frosting	42	4 oz	58	24
Vanilla pudding, instant, made with whole milk	40	½ cup	24	10
Vanilla wafers	77	6 cookies	18	14
Veal	[0]	4 oz	0	0
Vermicelli, white, cooked	35	1½ cups	44	16
W				
Waffles, Aunt Jemima®	76	1 4" waffle	13	10
Walnuts	[0]	1.75 oz	0	0
Water crackers	78	7 crackers	18	14
Watermelon, fresh	72	4 oz	6	4
Weet-Bix™, breakfast cereal	69	2 biscuits	17	12
Wheaties™, breakfast cereal	82	1 cup	21	17
Whiskey	[0]	1 oz	0	0
White bread	70	1 oz	14	10
White rice, instant, cooked 6 min	87	1 cup	42	36
White wine	[0]	3.5 oz	0	0
100% Whole Grain™ bread (Natural Ovens)	51	1 oz	13	7
Whole milk	31	8 oz	12	4
Whole-wheat bread	77	1 oz	12	9
Wonder™ white bread	80	1 oz	14	11
X				
Xylitol	8	1 Tbsp	10	1
Y				
Yam, peeled, cooked	37	5 oz	36	13
Yogurt, low-fat, wild strawberry	31	8 oz	34	11

[0] indicates that the food has so little carbohydrate that the GI value cannot be tested. The GL, therefore, is 0.

FOOD	GI Value	Nominal Serving Size	Net Carb per Serving	GL per Serving
Yogurt, low-fat, with fruit and artificial sweetener	14	8 oz	15	2
Yogurt, low-fat, with fruit and sugar	33	8 oz	35	12

[0] indicates that the food has so little carbohydrate that the GI value cannot be tested. The GL, therefore, is 0.

◀ 5 ▶

FOOD CATEGORY GI VALUES

THE FOLLOWING TABLE groups the foods we've tested by several categories, which include:

- ▶ bakery products
- ▶ beverages
- ▶ breads
- ▶ breakfast foods
- ▶ cookies
- ▶ crackers
- ▶ dairy products and alternatives
- ▶ fruits and fruit products
- ▶ grains
- ▶ infant formulas and baby foods
- ▶ legumes
- ▶ meal replacement products
- ▶ mixed meals and convenience foods
- ▶ noodles
- ▶ pasta

- ❥ protein foods
- ❥ snack foods and candy
- ❥ soups
- ❥ special dietary products
- ❥ sugars
- ❥ vegetables

Within each food category, we have grouped the foods in alphabetical order to help you choose low-GI foods within each category. You can also mix and match: If your favorite food has a high GI value, check out its glycemic load. If the GL is relatively low compared to other foods within that group, then you don't need to worry too much about its high GI value. If the food has both a high GI value and a high glycemic load (such as Instant white rice), cut down on the serving size or team it up with a very low-GI food, such as lentils.

We have included in the Food Categories Table all of the available data we've collected for these foods. In addition to GI values for foods sold within the United States, you'll also find GI values from all over the world, including Australia, Canada, New Zealand, Italy, Sweden, Japan, and China. We've also listed popular foods with low carbohydrate contents, such as meats, nuts, and alcoholic beverages. Their GI values are listed as [0].

NOTE: ▲ designates that a particular brand was not specified. ■ designates the average values of multiple studies.

FOOD	GI Value	Nominal Serving Size	Net Carb per Serving	GL per Serving
BAKERY PRODUCTS				
			[30 g = 1 oz]	
Cakes				
Angel food (Loblaw's, Canada)	67	50 g	29	19
Banana, made with sugar	47	80 g	38	18
Banana, made without sugar	55	80 g	29	16
Chocolate, made from packet mix with chocolate frosting (Betty Crocker)	38	111 g	52	20
Flan	65	70 g	48	31
Lamingtons (sponge dipped in chocolate and coconut)	87	50 g	29	25
Pound (Sara Lee)	54	53 g	28	15
Sponge, plain	46	63 g	36	17
Vanilla, made from mix with vanilla frosting (Betty Crocker)	42	111 g	58	24
Muffins and related foods				
Apple, made with sugar	44	60 g	29	13
Apple, made without sugar	48	60 g	19	9
Apple, oat, raisin, made from mix	54	50 g	26	14
Apricot, coconut, and honey, made from mix	60	50 g	26	16
Banana, oat, and honey, made from mix	65	50 g	26	17
Bran	60	57 g	24	15
Blueberry	59	57 g	29	17
Carrot	62	57 g	32	20
Chocolate butterscotch, made from packet mix	53	50 g	28	15
Crumpet	69	50 g	19	13
Cupcake, strawberry-iced	73	38 g	26	19

[0] indicates that the food has so little carbohydrate that the GI value cannot be tested. The GL, therefore, is 0. ▲ indicates brand not specified.

FOOD	GI Value	Nominal Serving Size	Net Carb per Serving	GL per Serving
Oatmeal, made from mix (Quaker Oats)	69	50 g	35	24
Pikelets, Golden brand (Tip Top)	85	40 g	21	18
Scones, plain, made from mix	92	25 g	9	8
Pastries				
Croissant	67	57 g	26	17
Doughnut, cake-type	76	47 g	23	17
Pastry	59	57 g	26	15

BEVERAGES

[30 mL = 1 oz; 250 mL = approx. 8 oz]

Alcoholic

Beer	[0]	250 mL	10	0
Brandy	[0]	30 mL	0	0
Gin	[0]	30 mL	0	0
Sherry	[0]	30 mL	0	0
Whiskey	[0]	30 mL	0	0
Wine, red	[0]	100 mL	0	0
Wine, white	[0]	100 mL	0	0

Juices

Apple juice, pure, unsweetened, reconstituted (Berri, Australia)	39	250 mL	25	10
Apple juice, unsweetened (USA)	40	250 mL	29	12
Apple juice, unsweetened (Allens, Canada)	41	250 mL	30	12
■ *average*	40	250 mL	28	11
Apple, pure, clear, unsweetened (Wild About Fruit, Australia)	44	250 mL	30	13
Apple, pure, cloudy, unsweetened (Wild About Fruit, Australia)	37	250 mL	28	10

[0] indicates that the food has so little carbohydrate that the GI value cannot be tested. The GL, therefore, is 0. ▲ indicates brand not specified.

FOOD	GI Value	Nominal Serving Size	Net Carb per Serving	GL per Serving
Carrot, freshly made (Sydney, Australia)	43	250 mL	23	10
Cranberry juice cocktail (Ocean Spray®, Australia)	52	250 mL	31	16
Cranberry juice cocktail (Ocean Spray®, USA)	68	250 mL	36	24
Cranberry juice drink (Ocean Spray®, UK)	56	250 mL	29	16
Grapefruit, unsweetened (Sunpac, Canada)	48	250 mL	22	11
Orange (Canada)	46	250 mL	26	12
Orange, reconstituted from frozen concentrate (USA)	57	250 mL	26	15
Orange, unsweetened, (Quelch®, Australia)	53	250 mL	18	9
■ average	52	250 mL	23	12
Pineapple, unsweetened (Dole, Canada)	46	250 mL	34	16
Tomato, canned, no added sugar (Berri, Australia)	38	250 mL	9	4

Powder drinks

FOOD	GI Value	Nominal Serving Size	Net Carb per Serving	GL per Serving
Build-Up™ with fiber (Nestlé)	41	250 mL	33	14
Complete Hot Chocolate mix with hot water (Nestlé)	51	250 mL	23	11
Hi-Pro energy drink mix, vanilla (Harrod)	36	250 mL	19	7
Malted milk in full-fat cow's milk (Nestlé, Australia)	45	250 mL	26	12
Milo™ (Nestlé, Auckland, New Zealand), in water	52	250 mL	16	9
Milo™ (Nestlé, Australia), in full-fat cow's milk	35	250 mL	25	9
Milo™ (Nestlé, Australia), in water	55	250 mL	16	9

[0] indicates that the food has so little carbohydrate that the GI value cannot be tested. The GL, therefore, is 0. ▲ indicates brand not specified.

FOOD	GI Value	Nominal Serving Size	Net Carb per Serving	GL per Serving
Milo™ (Nestlé, New Zealand), in full-fat cow's milk	36	250 mL	26	9
Milo™ (Nestlé, New Zealand), bottle	30	600 mL	64	19
Milo™ (Nestlé, New Zealand), petrapak	35	250 mL	31	11
Nutrimeal™, meal-replacement drink, Dutch Chocolate (Usana)	26	250 mL	17	4
Quik™, chocolate (Nestlé, Australia), in water	53	250 mL	7	4
Quik™, chocolate (Nestlé, Australia), in 1.5% milk	41	250 mL	11	5
Quik™, strawberry (Nestlé, Australia), in water	64	250 mL	8	5
Quik™, strawberry (Nestlé, Australia), in 1.5% milk	35	250 mL	12	4

Smoothies and shakes

FOOD	GI Value	Nominal Serving Size	Net Carb per Serving	GL per Serving
Smoothie, raspberry (Con Agra)	33	250 mL	41	14
Smoothie drink, soy, banana (So Natural)	30	250 mL	22	7
Smoothie drink, soy, chocolate hazelnut (So Natural)	34	250 mL	25	8
Up & Go, cocoa malt flavor (Sanitarium)	43	250 mL	26	11
Up & Go, original malt flavor (Sanitarium)	46	250 mL	24	11
Xpress, chocolate (So Natural, Australia)	39	250 mL	34	13
Yakult® (Yakult, Australia)	46	65 mL	12	6

Soft drinks

FOOD	GI Value	Nominal Serving Size	Net Carb per Serving	GL per Serving
Coca Cola®, soft drink (Australia)	53	250 mL	26	14
Coca Cola®, soft drink/soda (USA)	63	250 mL	26	16
Cordial, orange, reconstituted (Berri)	66	250 mL	20	13
Fanta®, orange soft drink (Australia)	68	250 mL	34	23
Lucozade®, original (sparkling glucose drink)	95	250 mL	42	40

[0] indicates that the food has so little carbohydrate that the GI value cannot be tested. The GL, therefore, is 0. ▲ indicates brand not specified.

FOOD	GI Value	Nominal Serving Size	Net Carb per Serving	GL per Serving
Solo™, lemon squash, soft drink (Australia)	58	250 mL	29	17

Sports drinks

Gatorade® (Australia)	78	250 mL	15	12
Isostar® (Switzerland)	70	250 mL	18	13
Sports Plus® (Australia)	74	250 mL	17	13
Sustagen Sport® (Australia)	43	250 mL	49	21

Yogurt drinks

Yogurt drink, reduced fat, Vaalia™, passionfruit (Pauls, Australia)	38	200 mL	29	11

BREADS

[30 g = 1 oz]

Barley flour

100% barley flour (Canada)	67	30 g	13	9
Sunflower and barley bread (Riga, Sydney, Australia)	57	30 g	11	6

Fruit

Bürgen™ Fruit loaf (Tip Top, Australia)	44	30 g	13	6
Continental fruit loaf, wheat bread with dried fruit (Australia)	47	30 g	15	7
Happiness™ (cinnamon, raisin, pecan bread) (Natural Ovens, USA)	63	30 g	14	9
Muesli bread, made from mix in bread oven (Con Agra Inc., USA)	54	30 g	12	7

Gluten-free

Gluten-free multigrain bread (Country Life Bakeries, Australia)	79	30 g	13	10

[0] indicates that the food has so little carbohydrate that the GI value cannot be tested. The GL, therefore, is 0. ▲ indicates brand not specified.

FOOD	GI Value	Nominal Serving Size	Net Carb per Serving	GL per Serving
Gluten-free white bread, sliced (gluten-free wheat starch) (UK)	80	30 g	15	12
Gluten-free white bread, unsliced (gluten-free wheat starch) (UK)	71	30 g	15	11
■ average	76	30 g	15	11
Gluten-free fiber-enriched, sliced (gluten-free wheat starch, soya bran) (UK)	76	30 g	13	10
Gluten-free fiber-enriched, unsliced (gluten-free wheat starch, soya bran) (UK)	69	30 g	13	9
■ average	73	30 g	13	9

Rice flour

FOOD	GI Value	Nominal Serving Size	Net Carb per Serving	GL per Serving
Rice bread, high-amylose Doongara rice (Pav's, Australia)	61	30 g	12	7
Rice bread, low-amylose Calrose rice (Pav's, Australia)	72	30 g	12	8

Rye flour

FOOD	GI Value	Nominal Serving Size	Net Carb per Serving	GL per Serving
Cocktail, sliced (Kasselar Food Products, Canada)	62	30 g	12	8
Cocktail, sliced (Kasselar Food Products, Canada)	55	30 g	12	7
Rye kernel, pumpernickel (Canada)	41	30 g	12	5
Rye kernel, pumpernickel (80% kernels) (Canada)	55	30 g	12	7
Whole grain pumpernickel (Holtzheuser Brothers Ltd., Canada)	46	30 g	11	5
■ average	50	30 g	12	6
Whole-wheat rye, average	58	30 g	14	8

Specialty rye

FOOD	GI Value	Nominal Serving Size	Net Carb per Serving	GL per Serving
Blackbread, Riga (Berzin's, Australia)	76	30 g	13	10

[0] indicates that the food has so little carbohydrate that the GI value cannot be tested. The GL, therefore, is 0. ▲ indicates brand not specified.

FOOD	GI Value	Nominal Serving Size	Net Carb per Serving	GL per Serving
Bürgen™ Dark/Swiss rye (Tip Top Bakeries, Australia)	65	30 g	10	7
Klosterbrot whole-wheat rye (Dimpflmeier, Canada)	67	30 g	13	9
Light rye (Silverstein's, Canada)	68	30 g	14	10
Linseed rye (Rudolph's, Canada)	55	30 g	13	7
Roggenbrot, Vogel's	59	30 g	14	8
Schinkenbrot, Riga (Berzin's, Australia)	86	30 g	14	12
Sourdough rye (average)	53	30 g	12	6
Volkornbrot, whole-wheat rye bread (Dimpflmeier, Canada)	56	30 g	13	7

Specialty wheat

FOOD	GI Value	Nominal Serving Size	Net Carb per Serving	GL per Serving
Bürgen® Mixed Grain (Tip Top, Australia)	49	30 g	11	6
Dürgen® Oat Bran & Honey Loaf with Barley (Tip Top, Australia)	49	40 g	13	7
Bürgen® Soy-Lin, kibbled soy (8%) and linseed (8%) loaf (Tip Top)	36	30 g	9	3
English Muffin™ bread (Natural Ovens, USA)	77	30 g	14	11
Healthy Choice™ Hearty 7 Grain (Con Agra, USA)	55	30 g	14	8
Healthy Choice™ Hearty 100% Whole Grain (Con Agra, USA)	62	30 g	14	9
Helga's™ Classic Seed Loaf (Quality Bakers, Australia)	68	30 g	14	9
Helga's™ traditional whole-wheat bread (Quality Bakers, Australia)	70	30 g	13	9
Holsum's sunflower and poppyseed	61	74 g	30	18
Holsum's whole meal and rye	63	74 g	28	18
Hunger Filler™, whole-grain bread (Natural Ovens, USA)	59	30 g	13	7

[0] indicates that the food has so little carbohydrate that the GI value cannot be tested. The GL, therefore, is 0. ▲ indicates brand not specified.

FOOD	GI Value	Nominal Serving Size	Net Carb per Serving	GL per Serving
Molenberg™ (Goodman Fielder, Auckland, New Zealand)	80	30 g	14	11
9-Grain Multi-Grain (Tip Top, Australia)	43	30 g	14	6
Nutty Natural™, whole grain (Natural Ovens, USA)	59	30 g	12	7
Performax™ (Country Life Bakeries, Australia)	38	30 g	13	5
Ploughman's™ whole grain, original recipe (Quality Bakers, Australia)	47	30 g	14	7
Ploughman's™ whole wheat, smooth milled (Quality Bakers, Australia)	64	30 g	13	9
Sourdough wheat (Australia)	54	30 g	14	8
Soy & Linseed, bread machine mix, (Con Agra, USA)	50	30 g	10	5
Stay Trim™, whole-grain (Natural Ovens, USA)	70	30 g	15	10
Sunflower & barley bread, Riga brand (Berzin's, Australia)	57	30 g	13	7
Vogel's Honey & Oats (Stevns & Co., Australia)	55	30 g	14	7
Vogel's Roggenbrot (Stevns & Co., Australia)	59	30 g	14	8
100% Whole Grain™ bread (Natural Ovens, USA)	51	30 g	13	7
Whole-wheat snack bread (Ryvita Co Ltd., UK)	74	30 g	22	16

Spelt

FOOD	GI Value	Nominal Serving Size	Net Carb per Serving	GL per Serving
Scalded spelt wheat kernel (Slovenia)	67	30 g	22	15
Spelt multigrain® (Pav's, Australia)	54	30 g	12	7
White spelt wheat (Slovenia)	74	30 g	23	17
Whole-wheat spelt wheat (Slovenia)	63	30 g	19	12

[0] indicates that the food has so little carbohydrate that the GI value cannot be tested. The GL, therefore, is 0. ▲ indicates brand not specified.

FOOD	GI Value	Nominal Serving Size	Net Carb per Serving	GL per Serving
Unleavened				
Amaranth : wheat (25:75) composite flour flatbread (India)	66	30 g	15	10
Amaranth : wheat (50:50) composite flour flatbread (India)	76	30 g	15	11
Lebanese, white (Seda Bakery, Australia)	75	30 g	16	12
Middle Eastern flatbread	97	30 g	16	15
Pita, white (Canada)	57	30 g	17	10
Wheat flour flatbread (India)	66	30 g	16	10
Wheat kernel				
Coarse wheat kernel, 80% intact kernels (Sweden)	52	30 g	20	10
White wheat flour				
Bagel, white, frozen (Canada)	72	70 g	35	25
Baguette, white, plain (France)	95	30 g	15	15
Bread stuffing, Paxo (Canada)	74	30 g	21	16
French baguette with butter and strawberry jam (France)	62	70 g	41	26
French baguette with chocolate spread (France)	72	70 g	37	27
Pain au lait (Pasquier, France)	63	60 g	32	20
White flour (Canada)	69	30 g	14	10
White flour (Canada)	71	30 g	14	10
White flour (Dempster's Corporate Foods Ltd., Canada)	71	30 g	14	10
White flour (South Africa)	71	30 g	13	9
White flour (USA)	70	30 g	14	10
White flour, Sunblest™ (Tip Top, Australia)	70	30 g	14	10
■ average	70	30 g	14	10

[0] indicates that the food has so little carbohydrate that the GI value cannot be tested. The GL, therefore, is 0. ▲ indicates brand not specified.

FOOD	GI Value	Nominal Serving Size	Net Carb per Serving	GL per Serving
White Turkish (Turkey)	87	30 g	17	15
White wheat flour, hard, toasted (Italian)	73	30 g	15	11
Wonder™, enriched white flour (average)	73	30 g	14	10

White wheat flour, fiber-enriched

White, high-fiber bread (average)	68	30 g	13	9

White wheat flour, resistant-starch-enriched

Fiber White™ (Nature's Fresh, New Zealand)	77	30 g	15	11
Wonderwhite™ (Buttercup, Australia)	80	30 g	14	11

White wheat flour with soluble fiber

White bread containing Eurylon® high-amylose maize starch (France)	42	30 g	19	8
White bread eaten with powdered dried seaweed	48	30 g	15	7
White bread eaten with vinegar as vinaigrette (Sweden)	45	30 g	15	7

Whole-wheat wheat flour

Whole-wheat flour (Canada)	66	30 g	12	8
Whole-wheat flour (Kenya)	87	30 g	13	11
Whole-wheat flour (South Africa)	75	30 g	13	9
Whole-wheat flour (Tip Top Bakeries, Australia)	78	30 g	12	9
Whole-wheat flour (USA)	73	30 g	14	10
Whole-wheat Turkish	49	30 g	16	8

[0] indicates that the food has so little carbohydrate that the GI value cannot be tested. The GL, therefore, is 0. ▲ indicates brand not specified.

FOOD	GI Value	Nominal Serving Size	Net Carb per Serving	GL per Serving

BREAKFAST FOODS

[30 g = 1 oz; 250 g = 1 cup]

Breakfast cereal bars

FOOD	GI Value	Nominal Serving Size	Net Carb per Serving	GL per Serving
Crunchy Nut Cornflakes™ bar (Kellogg's, Australia)	72	30 g	26	19
Fiber Plus™ bar (Uncle Toby's, Australia)	78	30 g	23	18
Fruity-Bix™ bar, fruit and nut (Sanitarium, Australia)	56	30 g	19	10
Fruity-Bix™ bar, wild berry (Sanitarium, Australia)	51	30 g	19	9
K-Time Just Right™ bar (Kellogg's, Australia)	72	30 g	24	17
K-Time Strawberry Crunch™ bar (Kellogg's, Australia)	77	30 g	25	19
Rice Bubble Treat™ bar (Kellogg's, Australia)	63	30 g	24	15
Sustain™ bar (Kellogg's, Australia)	57	30 g	25	14

Cooked cereals

FOOD	GI Value	Nominal Serving Size	Net Carb per Serving	GL per Serving
Cream of Wheat™ (Nabisco, Canada)	66	250 g	26	17
Cream of Wheat™, Instant (Nabisco, Canada)	74	250 g	30	22
Hot cereal, apple & cinnamon (Con Agra, USA)	37	30 g	22	8
Hot cereal, unflavored (Con Agra, USA)	25	30 g	19	5
Oatmeal, instant (USA)	75	250 g	23	17
Oatmeal/porridge (Australia)	58	250 g	21	12
Oatmeal/porridge (Canada)	49	250 g	23	11
Oatmeal/porridge (Canada)	62	250 g	23	14
Oatmeal/porridge (Canada)	69	250 g	23	16

[0] indicates that the food has so little carbohydrate that the GI value cannot be tested. The GL, therefore, is 0. ▲ indicates brand not specified.

FOOD	GI Value	Nominal Serving Size	Net Carb per Serving	GL per Serving
Oatmeal/porridge (Hubbards, New Zealand)	58	250 g	21	12
Oatmeal/porridge (Uncle Toby's, Australia)	42	250 g	21	9
Traditional porridge oats (Lowan, Australia)	51	250 g	21	11
■ average	58	250 g	22	13
One Minute Oats (Quaker Oats, Canada)	66	30 g (dry)	19	12
Quick Oats (Quaker Oats, Canada)	65	30 g (dry)	19	12
■ average	66	250 g	26	17
Ready-to-eat cereals				
All-Bran™ (Kellogg's, Australia)	30	30 g	15	4
All-Bran™ (Kellogg's, Canada)	51	30 g	23	9
All-Bran® (Kellogg's, USA)	38	30 g	23	9
■ average	40	30 g	21	9
All-Bran Fruit 'n' Oats™ (Kellogg's, Australia)	39	30 g	17	7
All-Bran Soy 'n' Fiber™ (Kellogg's, Australia)	33	30 g	14	4
Alpen Muesli (Wheatabix, France)	55	30 g	19	10
Amaranth, popped, with milk (India)	97	30 g	19	18
Bran Buds with psyllium (Kellogg's, Canada)	47	30 g	12	6
Bran Buds™ (Kellogg's, Canada)	58	30 g	12	7
Bran Chex™ (Nabisco, Canada)	58	30 g	19	11
Bran Flakes™ (Kellogg's, Australia)	74	30 g	18	13
Cheerios™ (General Mills, Canada)	74	30 g	20	15
Chocapic™ (Nestlé, France)	84	30 g	25	21
Coco Pops™ (Kellogg's, Australia)	77	30 g	26	20

[0] indicates that the food has so little carbohydrate that the GI value cannot be tested. The GL, therefore, is 0. ▲ indicates brand not specified.

FOOD	GI Value	Nominal Serving Size	Net Carb per Serving	GL per Serving
Corn Bran™ (Quaker Oats, Canada)	75	30 g	20	15
Corn Chex™ (Nabisco, Canada)	83	30 g	25	21
Corn Pops™ (Kellogg's, Australia)	80	30 g	26	21
Cornflakes, Crunchy Nut™ (Kellogg's, Australia)	72	30 g	24	17
Cornflakes, high fiber (Presidents Choice, Canada)	74	30 g	23	17
Cornflakes™ (Kellogg's, Australia)	77	30 g	25	20
Cornflakes™ (Kellogg's, Canada)	83	30 g	25	22
Cornflakes™ (Kellogg's, New Zealand)	72	30 g	25	18
Corn Flakes™ (Kellogg's, USA)	92	30 g	26	24
■ *average*	81	30 g	26	21
Crispix™ (Kellogg's, Canada)	87	30 g	25	22
Energy Mix™ (Quaker, France)	80	30 g	24	19
Froot Loops™ (Kellogg's, Australia)	69	30 g	26	18
Frosties™, sugar-coated cornflakes (Kellogg's, Australia)	55	30 g	26	15
Fruitful Lite™ (Hubbards, New Zealand)	61	30 g	20	12
Fruity-Bix™, berry (Sanitarium, New Zealand)	113	30 g	22	25
Golden Grahams™ (General Mills, Canada)	71	30 g	25	18
Golden Wheats™ (Kellogg's, Australia)	71	30 g	23	16
Good Start™, muesli wheat biscuits (Sanitarium, Australia)	68	30 g	20	14
Grapenuts™ (Kraft, USA)	75	30 g	22	16
Grapenuts™ (Post, Kraft, Canada)	67	30 g	19	13
■ *average*	71	30 g	21	15
Grapenuts™ Flakes (Post, Canada)	80	30 g	22	17

[0] indicates that the food has so little carbohydrate that the GI value cannot be tested. The GL, therefore, is 0. ▲ indicates brand not specified.

FOOD	GI Value	Nominal Serving Size	Net Carb per Serving	GL per Serving
Guardian™ (Kellogg's, Australia)	37	30 g	12	5
Healthwise™ for bowel health (Uncle Toby's, Australia)	66	30 g	18	12
Healthwise™ for heart health (Uncle Toby's, Australia)	48	30 g	19	9
Hi-Bran Weet-Bix™ with soy and linseed (Sanitarium, Australia)	57	30 g	16	9
Hi-Bran Weet-Bix™, wheat biscuits (Sanitarium, Australia)	61	30 g	17	10
Honey Goldies™ (Kellogg's, Australia)	72	30 g	21	15
Honey Rice Bubbles™ (Kellogg's, Australia)	77	30 g	27	20
Honey Smacks™ (Kellogg's, Australia)	71	30 g	23	16
Just Right Just Grains™ (Kellogg's, Australia)	62	30 g	23	14
Just Right™ (Kellogg's, Australia)	60	30 g	22	13
Komplete™ (Kellogg's, Australia)	48	30 g	21	10
Life™ (Quaker Oats Co., Canada)	66	30 g	25	16
Lite-Bix™, plain, no added sugar (Sanitarium, Australia)	70	30 g	20	14
Mini Wheats™, blackcurrant (Kellogg's, Australia)	72	30 g	21	15
Mini Wheats™, whole wheat (Kellogg's, Australia)	58	30 g	21	12
Muesli (Canada)	66	30 g	24	16
Muesli, gluten-free (Freedom Foods, Australia)	39	30 g	19	7
Muesli, Lite (Sanitarium, New Zealand)	54	30 g	18	10
Muesli, Natural (Sanitarium, Australia)	40	30 g	19	8
Muesli, Natural (Sanitarium, New Zealand)	57	30 g	19	11
Muesli, No Name (Sunfresh, Canada)	60	30 g	18	11
Muesli, Swiss Formula (Uncle Toby's, Australia)	56	30 g	16	9

[0] indicates that the food has so little carbohydrate that the GI value cannot be tested. The GL, therefore, is 0. ▲ indicates brand not specified.

FOOD	GI Value	Nominal Serving Size	Net Carb per Serving	GL per Serving
Muesli, toasted (Purina, Australia)	43	30 g	17	7
Nutrigrain™ (Kellogg's, Australia)	66	30 g	15	10
Oat bran Weet-Bix™ (Sanitarium, Australia)	57	30 g	20	11
Oat 'n' Honey Bake™ (Kellogg's, Australia)	77	30 g	17	13
Oat bran, raw (Quaker Oats, Canada)	50	10 g	5	2
Oat bran, raw	59	10 g	5	3
■ *average*	55	10 g	5	3
Pro Stars™ (General Mills, Canada)	71	30 g	24	17
Puffed Wheat (Quaker Oats, Canada)	67	30 g	20	13
Puffed Wheat (Sanitarium, Australia)	80	30 g	21	17
■ *average*	74	30 g	21	16
Raisin Bran™ (Kellogg's, USA)	61	30 g	19	12
Red River Cereal (Maple Leaf Mills, Canada)	49	30 g	22	11
Rice Bran, extruded (Rice Growers, Australia)	19	30 g	14	3
Rice Bubbles™ (Kellogg's, Australia) (average)	87	30 g	26	22
Rice Chex™ (Nabisco, Canada)	89	30 g	26	23
Rice Krispies™ (Kellogg's, Canada)	82	30 g	26	21
Shredded Wheat (Canada)	67	30 g	20	13
Shredded Wheat™ (Nabisco, Canada)	83	30 g	20	17
■ *average*	75	30 g	20	15
Soy Tasty™ (Sanitarium, Australia)	60	30 g	20	12

[0] indicates that the food has so little carbohydrate that the GI value cannot be tested. The GL, therefore, is 0. ▲ indicates brand not specified.

FOOD	GI Value	Nominal Serving Size	Net Carb per Serving	GL per Serving
Soytana™ (Vogel's, Australia)	49	45 g	25	12
Special K™ (Kellogg's, Australia)	54	30 g	21	11
Special K™ (Kellogg's, France)	84	30 g	24	20
Special K™ (Kellogg's, USA)	69	30 g	21	14
Sultana Bran™ (Kellogg's, Australia)	73	30 g	19	14
Sultana Goldies™ (Kellogg's, Australia)	65	30 g	21	13
Sustain™ (Kellogg's, Australia)	68	30 g	22	15
Team™ (Nabisco, Canada)	82	30 g	22	17
Thank Goodness™ (Hubbards, New Zealand)	65	30 g	23	15
Total™ (General Mills, Canada)	76	30 g	22	17
Ultra-bran™ (Vogel's, Australia)	41	30 g	13	5
Weetabix™ (Weetabix, Canada)	74	30 g	22	16
Weetabix™ (Weetabix, Canada)	75	30 g	22	16
Wheat-bites™ (Uncle Toby's, Australia)	72	30 g	25	18
Whole-wheat Goldies™ (Kellogg's, Australia)	70	30 g	20	14

Grain products

FOOD	GI Value	Nominal Serving Size	Net Carb per Serving	GL per Serving
Pancakes, prepared from shake mix	67	70 g	23	15
Pancakes, buckwheat, gluten-free, made from packet mix (Orgran)	102	77 g	22	22
Waffles, Aunt Jemima®	76	35 g	13	10

COOKIES

[30 g = 1 oz]

FOOD	GI Value	Nominal Serving Size	Net Carb per Serving	GL per Serving
Arrowroot (McCormick's, Canada)	63	25 g	20	13
Arrowroot plus (McCormick's, Canada)	62	25 g	18	11
Milk Arrowroot™ (Arnotts, Australia)	69	25 g	18	12
■ average	65	25 g	19	12

[0] indicates that the food has so little carbohydrate that the GI value cannot be tested. The GL, therefore, is 0. ▲ indicates brand not specified.

FOOD	GI Value	Nominal Serving Size	Net Carb per Serving	GI per Serving
Barquette Abricot (LU, France)	71	40 g	32	23
Bebe Dobre Rano Chocolate (LU, Czech Republic)	57	50 g	33	19
Bebe Dobre Rano Honey and Hazelnuts (LU, Czech Republic)	51	50 g	34	17
Bebe Jemne Susenky (LU, Czech Republic)	67	25 g	20	14
Digestives (Canada)	59	25 g	16	10
Digestives, gluten-free (Nutricia, UK)	58	25 g	17	10
Evergreen met Krenten (LU, Netherlands)	66	38 g	21	14
Golden Fruit (Griffin's, New Zealand)	77	25 g	17	13
Graham Wafers (Christie Brown, Canada)	74	25 g	18	14
Gran'Dia Banana, Oats and Honey (LU, Brazil)	28	30 g	23	6
Grany en-cas Abricot (LU, France)	55	30 g	16	9
Grany en-cas Fruits des bois (LU, France)	50	30 g	14	7
Grany Rush Apricot (LU, Netherlands)	62	30 g	20	12
Highland Oatcakes (Walker's, Scotland)	57	25 g	15	8
Highland Oatmeal™ (Westons, Australia)	55	25 g	18	10
LU P'tit Déjeuner Chocolat (LU, France)	42	50 g	34	14
LU P'tit Déjeuner Miel et Pépites Chocolat (LU, France)	49	50 g	35	17
Maltmeal wafer (Griffin's, New Zealand)	50	25 g	17	9
Morning Coffee™ (Arnotts, Australia)	79	25 g	19	15
Nutrigrain Fruits des bois (Kellogg's, France)	57	35 g	23	13
Oatmeal (Canada)	54	25 g	17	9
Oro (Saiwa, Italy) (average)	64	40 g	32	20
Petit LU Normand (LU, France)	51	25 g	19	10

[0] indicates that the food has so little carbohydrate that the GI value cannot be tested. The GL, therefore, is 0. ▲ indicates brand not specified.

FOOD	GI Value	Nominal Serving Size	Net Carb per Serving	GL per Serving
Petit LU Roussillon (LU, France)	48	25 g	18	9
Prince Energie+ (LU, France)	73	25 g	17	13
Prince fourré chocolat (LU, France) (average)	52	65 g	30	16
Prince Meganana Chocolate (LU, Spain)	49	50 g	36	18
Prince Petit Déjeuner Vanille (LU, France and Spain)	45	50 g	36	16
Rich Tea (Canada)	55	25 g	19	10
Sablé des Flandres (LU, France)	57	20 g	15	8
Shortbread (Arnotts, Australia)	64	25 g	16	10
Shredded Wheatmeal™ (Arnotts, Australia)	62	25 g	18	11
Snack Right Fruit Slice (97% fat-free) (Arnotts, Australia)	48	25 g	19	9
Thé (LU, France)	41	20 g	16	6
Vanilla Wafers (Christie Brown, Canada)	77	25 g	18	14
Véritable Petit Beurre (LU, France)	51	25 g	18	9

CRACKERS

[25 g = 0.8 oz]

FOOD	GI Value	Nominal Serving Size	Net Carb per Serving	GL per Serving
Breton wheat crackers (Dare Foods, Canada)	67	25 g	14	10
Corn Thins, puffed corn cakes, gluten-free (Real Foods, Australia)	87	25 g	20	18
Cream cracker (LU, Brazil)	65	25 g	17	11
High-calcium cracker (Danone, Malaysia)	52	25 g	17	9
Jatz™, plain salted cracker biscuits (Arnotts, Australia)	55	25 g	17	10
Kavli™ Norwegian Crispbread (Players, Australia)	71	25 g	16	12
Melba Toast, Old London (Best Foods, Canada)	70	30 g	23	16

[0] indicates that the food has so little carbohydrate that the GI value cannot be tested. The GL, therefore, is 0. ▲ indicates brand not specified.

FOOD	GI Value	Nominal Serving Size	Net Carb per Serving	GL per Serving
Premium Soda Crackers (Christie Brown, Canada)	74	25 g	17	12
Puffed Crispbread (Westons, Australia)	81	25 g	19	15
Puffed rice cakes (Rice Growers, Australia)	82	25 g	21	17
Rye crispbread (Canada)	63	25 g	16	10
Rye crispbread, high fiber (Ryvita, UK)	59	25 g	15	9
Rye crispbread (Ryvita, UK)	63	25 g	18	11
Ryvita™ (Canada)	69	25 g	16	11
■ *average*	64	25 g	16	11
Sao™, plain square crackers (Arnotts, Australia)	70	25 g	17	12
Stoned Wheat Thins (Christie Brown, Canada)	67	25 g	17	12
Water cracker (Canada)	63	25 g	18	11
Water cracker (Arnotts, Australia)	78	25 g	18	14
■ *average*	71	25 g	18	13
Vita-wheat™, original, crispbread (Arnotts, Australia)	55	25 g	19	10

DAIRY PRODUCTS AND ALTERNATIVES

[**50 g = 1.7 oz; 100 g = 3.3 oz; 250 g = approx. 8 oz**]

Custard

Custard, homemade (Australia)	43	100 g	17	7
No Bake Egg Custard (Nestlé, Australia)	35	100 g	17	6

[0] indicates that the food has so little carbohydrate that the GI value cannot be tested. The GL, therefore, is 0. ▲ indicates brand not specified.

FOOD	GI Value	Nominal Serving Size	Net Carb per Serving	GL per Serving
TRIM™, reduced-fat custard (Pauls, Australia)	37	100 g	15	6
■ average	38	100 g	16	6

Frozen desserts

Vitari, wild berry, non-dairy, frozen dessert (Nestlé, Australia)	59	100 g	21	12

Ice cream

1.2% fat, Prestige Light vanilla (Norco, Australia)	47	50 g	10	5
1.4% fat, Prestige Light toffee (Norco, Australia)	37	50 g	14	5
7.1% fat, Prestige golden macadamia (Norco, Australia)	37	50 g	9	3
French vanilla, 16% fat (Sara Lee, Australia)	38	50 g	9	3
Regular (average)	61	50 g	13	8
Ultra chocolate, 15% fat (Sara Lee, Australia)	37	50 g	9	4
Vanilla (Peter's, Australia)	50	50 g	6	3

Milk

Condensed, sweetened (Nestlé, Australia)	61	50 mL	136	33
Low-fat, chocolate, with aspartame, Lite White™ (Australia)	24	250 mL	15	3
Low-fat, chocolate, with sugar, Lite White™ (Australia)	34	250 mL	26	9
Skim (Canada)	32	250 mL	13	4
Whole (average)	27	250 mL	12	3

Mousse

Butterscotch, 1.9% fat (Nestlé, Australia)	36	50 g	10	4

[0] indicates that the food has so little carbohydrate that the GI value cannot be tested. The GL, therefore, is 0. ▲ indicates brand not specified.

FOOD	GI Value	Nominal Serving Size	Net Carb per Serving	GI per Serving
Chocolate, 2% fat (Nestlé, Australia)	31	50 g	11	3
French vanilla, 2% fat (Nestlé, Australia)	42	100 g	6	3
Hazelnut, 2.4% fat (Nestlé, Australia)	36	50 g	10	4
Mango, 1.8% fat (Nestlé, Australia)	33	50 g	11	4
Mixed berry, 2.2% fat (Nestlé, Australia)	36	50 g	10	4
Strawberry, 2.3% fat (Nestlé, Australia)	32	50 g	10	3
■ *average*	34	50 g	10	4

Pudding

FOOD	GI Value	Nominal Serving Size	Net Carb per Serving	GI per Serving
Instant, chocolate, made from powder and milk (White Wings, Australia)	47	100 g	16	7
Instant, vanilla, made from powder and milk (White Wings, Australia)	40	100 g	16	6
■ *average*	44	100 g	16	7

Soy milk

FOOD	GI Value	Nominal Serving Size	Net Carb per Serving	GI per Serving
Reduced fat, Light (So Natural, Australia)	44	250 g	17	8
Whole, Calciforte (So Natural, Australia)	36	250 g	18	6
Whole, Original (So Natural, Australia)	44	250 g	17	8
■ *average*	32	250 g	23	7
Up & Go™, cocoa malt flavor (Sanitarium, Australia)	43	250 g	26	11
Up & Go™, original malt flavor (Sanitarium, Australia)	46	250 g	24	11
■ *average*	45	250 g	25	11
Xpress™, chocolate (So Natural, Australia)	39	250 g	34	13

[0] indicates that the food has so little carbohydrate that the GI value cannot be tested. The GL, therefore, is 0. ▲ indicates brand not specified.

FOOD	GI Value	Nominal Serving Size	Net Carb per Serving	GL per Serving
Soy yogurt				
Peach and mango, 2% fat, with sugar (So Natural, Australia)	50	200 g	26	13
Tofu-based frozen dessert, chocolate (USA)	115	50 g	9	10
Yogurt				
Low-fat, fruit, with aspartame, Ski™ (Dairy Farmers, Australia)	14	200 g	13	2
Low-fat, fruit, with sugar, Ski™ (Dairy Farmers, Australia)	33	200 g	31	10
Low-fat (0.9%), fruit, wild strawberry, Ski d'lite™ (Dairy Farmers, Australia)	31	200 g	30	9
Diet Vaalia™, vanilla (Pauls, Australia)	23	200 g	13	3
Nonfat, French vanilla, with sugar, Vaalia™ (Pauls, Australia)	40	150 g	27	10
Nonfat, mango, Vaalia™, with sugar (Pauls, Australia)	39	150 g	25	10
Nonfat, strawberry, Vaalia™, with sugar (Pauls, Australia)	38	150 g	22	8
Nonfat, wild berry, Vaalia™, with sugar (Pauls, Australia)	23	200 g	13	3
Reduced fat, Vaalia™, apricot & mango (Pauls, Australia)	26	200 g	30	8
Reduced fat, Vaalia™, French vanilla (Pauls, Australia)	26	200 g	10	3
Reduced fat, Extra-Lite™, strawberry (Pauls, Australia)	28	200 g	33	9
■ *average*	27	200 g	24	7
Yogurt, type ▲ (Canada)	36	200 g	9	3

[0] indicates that the food has so little carbohydrate that the GI value cannot be tested. The GL, therefore, is 0. ▲ indicates brand not specified.

FOOD	GI Value	Nominal Serving Size	Net Carb per Serving	GL per Serving
FRUIT and FRUIT PRODUCTS				
			[60 g = 2 oz]	
Apple, Braeburn (New Zealand)	32	120 g	13	4
Apple, Golden Delicious (Canada)	39	120 g	16	6
Apple, ▲ (Canada)	34	120 g	16	5
Apple, ▲ (Denmark)	28	120 g	13	4
Apple, ▲ (Italy)	44	120 g	13	6
Apple, ▲ (USA)	40	120 g	16	6
■ *average*	38	120 g	15	6
Apple, dried (Australia)	29	60 g	34	10
Apricots, canned in light syrup (Riviera, Canada)	64	120 g	19	12
Apricots, dried (Australia)	30	60 g	27	8
Apricots, dried (Wasco, Canada)	32	60 g	30	10
Apricots, fresh (Italy)	57	120 g	9	5
■ *average*	31	60 g	28	9
Apricot fruit spread (Glen Ewin, Australia)	55	30 g	13	7
Banana (Canada)	46	120 g	25	12
Banana (Canada)	58	120 g	25	15
Banana (Canada)	62	120 g	25	16
Banana (Italy)	58	120 g	23	13
Banana (South Africa)	70	120 g	23	16
Banana, over-ripe (yellow flecked with brown) (USA)	48	120 g	25	12
Banana, over-ripe (Denmark)	52	120 g	20	11
Banana, ripe (all yellow) (USA)	51	120 g	25	13

[0] indicates that the food has so little carbohydrate that the GI value cannot be tested. The GL, therefore, is 0. ▲ indicates brand not specified.

FOOD	GI Value	Nominal Serving Size	Net Carb per Serving	GL per Serving
Banana, slightly under-ripe (yellow with green sections) (USA)	42	120 g	25	11
Banana, under-ripe (Denmark)	30	120 g	21	6
■ *average*	52	120 g	24	12
Breadfruit (*Artocarpus altilis*), raw (Australia)	68	120 g	27	18
Cantaloupe, fresh (Australia)	65	120 g	6	4
Cherries, fresh, ▲ (Canada)	22	120 g	12	3
Chico (*Zapota zapotilla coville*), raw (Philippines)	40	120 g	29	12
Custard apple, fresh, flesh only (Australia)	54	120 g	19	10
Dates, dried (Australia)	103	60 g	40	42
Figs, dried, tenderized (Dessert Maid, Australia)	61	60 g	26	16
Fruit Cocktail, canned (Delmonte, Canada)	55	120 g	16	9
Grapefruit, fresh (Canada)	25	120 g	11	3
Grapes, ▲ (Canada)	43	120 g	17	7
Grapes, ▲ (Italy)	49	120 g	19	9
■ *average*	46	120 g	18	8
Grapes, black, Waltham Cross (Australia)	59	120 g	18	11
Kiwi, Hayward (New Zealand)	47	120 g	12	5
Kiwi (Australia)	58	120 g	12	7
■ *average*	53	120 g	12	6
Lychee, canned in syrup and drained, Narcissus brand (China)	79	120 g	20	16

[0] indicates that the food has so little carbohydrate that the GI value cannot be tested. The GL, therefore, is 0. ▲ indicates brand not specified.

FOOD	GI Value	Nominal Serving Size	Net Carb per Serving	GL per Serving
Mango (*Mangifera indica*) (Philippines)	41	120 g	20	8
Mango (*Mangifera indica*) (Australia)	51	120 g	15	8
Mango, ripe (*Mangifera indica*) (India)	60	120 g	15	9
■ *average*	51	120 g	17	8
Mango, Frutia™ (Weis, Australia)	42	100 g	23	10
Marmalade, orange (Australia)	48	30 g	20	9
Oranges, ▲ (Canada)	40	120 g	11	4
Oranges, ▲ (Canada)	51	120 g	11	6
Oranges, ▲ (Denmark)	31	120 g	11	3
Oranges, ▲ (Italy)	48	120 g	11	5
Oranges, ▲ (South Africa)	33	120 g	10	3
Oranges (Sunkist, USA)	48	120 g	11	5
■ *average*	42	120 g	11	5
Papaya/paw paw, fresh (*Carica papaya*) (Australia)	56	120 g	8	5
Papaya/paw paw, ripe, fresh (India)	60	120 g	29	17
Papaya, fresh (*Carica papaya*) (Philippines)	60	120 g	15	9
■ *average*	59	120 g	17	10
Peach, fresh (Canada)	28	120 g	13	4
Peach, fresh (Italy)	56	120 g	8	5
■ *average*	42	120 g	11	5
Peach, canned in natural juice (Ardmona, Australia)	30	120 g	11	3
Peach, canned in natural juice (SPC, Australia)	45	120 g	11	5
■ *average*	38	120 g	11	4

[0] indicates that the food has so little carbohydrate that the GI value cannot be tested. The GL, therefore, is 0. ▲ indicates brand not specified.

FOOD	GI Value	Nominal Serving Size	Net Carb per Serving	GL per Serving
Peach, canned in heavy syrup (Letona, Australia)	58	120 g	15	9
Peach, canned in light syrup (Delmonte, Canada)	52	120 g	18	9
Peach, canned in reduced-sugar syrup (SPC, Australia)	62	120 g	17	11
Pear, fresh, ▲ (Canada)	33	120 g	13	4
Pear, Winter Nellis, fresh (New Zealand)	34	120 g	12	4
Pear, Bartlett, fresh (Canada)	41	120 g	8	3
Pear, fresh, ▲ (Italy)	42	120 g	11	4
■ average	38	120 g	11	4
Pear halves, canned in reduced-sugar syrup (SPC Lite, Australia)	25	120 g	14	4
Pear halves, canned in natural juice (SPC, Australia)	43	120 g	13	5
Pear, canned in pear juice, Bartlett (Delmonte, Canada)	44	120 g	11	5
Pineapple, fresh (Australia)	66	120 g	10	6
Pineapple (*Ananas comosus*), raw (Philippines)	51	120 g	16	8
■ average	59	120 g	13	7
Plum, fresh, ▲ (Canada)	24	120 g	14	3
Plum, fresh, ▲ (Italy)	53	120 g	11	6
■ average	39	120 g	12	5
Prunes, pitted (Sunsweet, USA)	29	60 g	33	10
Raisins (Canada)	64	60 g	44	28
Raisins/sultanas	56	60 g	45	25

[0] indicates that the food has so little carbohydrate that the GI value cannot be tested. The GL, therefore, is 0. ▲ indicates brand not specified.

FOOD	GI Value	Nominal Serving Size	Net Carb per Serving	GL per Serving
Strawberries, fresh (Australia)	40	120 g	3	1
Strawberry jam	51	30 g	20	10
Watermelon, fresh (Australia)	72	120 g	6	4

GRAINS

[150 g = 5 oz]

Amaranth

Amaranth (*Amaranthus esculentum*) popped, with milk	97	30 g	22	21

Barley

Barley, cracked (Malthouth, Tunisia)	50	150 g	42	21
Barley, pearled (average)	25	150 g	42	11
Barley, rolled (Australia)	66	50 g (dry)	38	25

Buckwheat

Buckwheat (average)	54	150 g	30	16
Buckwheat groats, cooked 12 min (Sweden)	45	150 g	30	13

Corn

Cornmeal, cooked in salted water 2 min (Canada)	68	150 g	13	9
Cornmeal + margarine (Canada)	69	150 g	12	9
■ *average*	69	150 g	13	9
Sweet, "Honey & Pearl" variety (New Zealand)	37	150 g	30	11
Sweet, on the cob, cooked 20 min (Australia)	48	150 g	30	14
Sweet (Canada)	59	150 g	33	20
Sweet (USA)	60	150 g	33	20

[0] indicates that the food has so little carbohydrate that the GI value cannot be tested. The GL, therefore, is 0. ▲ indicates brand not specified.

FOOD	GI Value	Nominal Serving Size	Net Carb per Serving	GL per Serving
Sweet (South Africa)	62	150 g	33	20
■ average	53	150 g	32	17
Sweet, canned, diet-pack (USA)	46	150 g	28	13
Sweet, frozen, reheated in microwave (Canada)	47	150 g	33	16

Couscous

Couscous, cooked 5 min (average)	65	150 g	35	23

Millet

Millet, cooked (Canada)	71	150 g	36	25

Rice

Arborio, risotto rice, cooked (Sun Rice, Australia)	69	150 g	43	29
Basmati, cooked (Mahatma, Australia)	58	150 g	42	24
Basmati, precooked, Uncle Ben's Express® (UK)	57	150 g	41	24
Basmati, quick-cooking, Uncle Ben's® Superior (Belgium)	60	150 g	38	23
Broken rice (Lion Foods, Thailand)	86	150	43	37
Brown (Canada)	66	150 g	33	21
Brown, steamed (USA)	50	150 g	33	16
Brown (*Oriza sativa*), cooked (South India)	50	150 g	33	16
■ average	55	150 g	33	18
Brown, Calrose (Rice Growers, Australia)	87	150 g	40	35
Brown, Doongara, high-amylose (Rice Growers, Australia)	66	150 g	37	24

[0] indicates that the food has so little carbohydrate that the GI value cannot be tested. The GL, therefore, is 0. ▲ indicates brand not specified.

FOOD	GI Value	Nominal Serving Size	Net Carb per Serving	GL per Serving
Brown, Pelde (Rice Growers, Australia)	76	150 g	38	29
Brown, parboiled, cooked 20 min, Uncle Ben's Natur-reis® (Belgium)	64	150 g	36	23
Brown, Sunbrown Quick™ (Rice Growers, Australia)	80	150 g	38	31
Cajun Style, Uncle Ben's® (Effem Foods, Canada)	51	150 g	37	19
Garden Style, Uncle Ben's® (Effem Foods, Canada)	55	150 g	37	21
Glutinous (sticky) rice (Thailand)	98	150 g	32	31
Instant, white, cooked 1 min (Canada)	46	150 g	42	19
Instant, white, cooked 6 min (Trice brand, Australia)	87	150 g	42	36
Puffed, white, cooked 5 min, Uncle Ben's Snabbris® (Belgium)	74	150 g	42	31
■ *average*	69	150 g	42	29
Instant Doongara, white, cooked 5 min (Rice Growers, Australia)	94	150 g	42	35
Jasmine rice (Thailand)	109	150 g	42	46
Gem long grain (Dainty, Canada)	58	150 g	40	24
Long grain (Uncle Ben's®, New Zealand)	56	150 g	43	24
Long grain, cooked 15 min	58	150 g	40	23
Long grain, cooked 15 min (Mahatma, Australia)	50	150 g	43	21
Long grain, cooked 5 min (Canada)	41	150 g	40	16
Long grain, cooked 7 min (Star, Canada)	64	150 g	40	26
Long grain, cooked 25 min (Surinam)	56	150 g	43	24
■ *average*	55	150 g	41	23
Long Grain and Wild, Uncle Ben's® (Effem Foods, Canada)	54	150 g	37	20

[0] indicates that the food has so little carbohydrate that the GI value cannot be tested. The GL, therefore, is 0. ▲ indicates brand not specified.

FOOD	GI Value	Nominal Serving Size	Net Carb per Serving	GL per Serving
Long grain, microwaved 2 min (Express Rice, Masterfoods, UK)	52	150 g	37	19
Long grain, parboiled 10 min cooking time (Uncle Ben's®, Belgium)	68	150 g	37	25
Long grain, parboiled, 20 min cooking time (Uncle Ben's®, Belgium)	75	150 g	37	28
Mexican Fast and Fancy, Uncle Ben's® (Effem Foods, Canada)	58	150 g	37	22
Parboiled (Canada)	48	150 g	36	18
Parboiled (USA)	72	150 g	36	26
Parboiled, converted, white, Uncle Ben's® (Canada)	45	150 g	36	16
Parboiled, converted, white, cooked 20–30 min, Uncle Ben's® (USA)	38	150 g	36	14
Parboiled, converted, white, long grain, cooked 20–30 min, Uncle Ben's® (USA)	50	150 g	36	18
Parboiled, cooked 12 min (Denmark)	43	150 g	36	15
Parboiled, long grain, cooked 5 min (Canada)	38	150 g	36	14
Parboiled, long grain, cooked 10 min (USA)	61	150 g	36	22
Parboiled, long grain, cooked 15 min (Canada)	47	150 g	36	17
Parboiled, long grain, cooked 25 min (Canada)	46	150 g	36	17
■ average	47	150 g	36	17
Parboiled, low-amylose, Bangladeshi variety BR2, (12% amylose)	51	150 g	38	19
Parboiled, low-amylose, Sungold (Rice Growers, Australia)	87	150 g	39	34

[0] indicates that the food has so little carbohydrate that the GI value cannot be tested. The GL, therefore, is 0. ▲ indicates brand not specified.

FOOD	GI Value	Nominal Serving Size	Net Carb per Serving	GL per Serving
Parboiled, high-amylose (28%), Doongara (Rice Growers, Australia)	50	150 g	42	21
Parboiled, high-amylose, Bangladeshi variety BR16 (28% amylose)	35	150 g	37	13
Parboiled, high-amylose, Bangladeshi variety BR16 pressure parboiled (27% amylose)	27	150 g	41	11
Parboiled, high-amylose, Bangladeshi variety BR16 traditional method (27% amylose)	32	150 g	38	12
Parboiled, high-amylose, Bangladeshi variety BR4 (27% amylose)	33	150 g	38	13
■ *average*	35	150 g	39	14
Saskatchewan wild rice (Canada)	57	150 g	32	18
White, high-amylose, Bangladeshi variety BR16 (28% amylose)	37	150 g	39	14
White, high-amylose, Bangladeshi variety BR16, long-grain (27% amylose)	39	150 g	39	15
■ *average*	38	150 g	39	15
White, high-amylose, Doongara (Rice Growers, Australia) (average)	56	150 g	42	24
White, high-amylose, Koshikari (Japonica), short-grain (Japan)	48	150 g	42	20
White, low-amylose, cooked (Turkey)	139	150 g	43	60
White, low-amylose, medium grain, Calrose, cooked (Rice Growers, Australia)	83	150 g	43	36
White, low-amylose, Pelde, (Rice Growers, Australia)	93	150 g	43	40
White, low-amylose, Sungold, Pelde, parboiled (Rice Growers, Australia)	87	150 g	43	37
White, low-amylose, Waxy (0–2% amylose) (Rice Growers, Australia)	88	150 g	43	38
White (*Oryza sativa*), cooked (India)	69	150 g	43	30

[0] indicates that the food has so little carbohydrate that the GI value cannot be tested. The GL, therefore, is 0. ▲ indicates brand not specified.

FOOD	GI Value	Nominal Serving Size	Net Carb per Serving	GL per Serving
White, Type ▲ (France)	45	150 g	30	14
White, Type ▲ (India)	48	150 g	38	18
White, Type ▲ (France)	52	150 g	36	19
White, Type ▲ (Pakistan)	69	150 g	38	26
White, Type ▲ (Canada)	60	150 g	42	25
White, Type ▲, cooked in salted water (India)	72	150 g	38	27
White, Type ▲, cooked 13 min (Italy)	102	150 g	30	31
White, Type ▲ (Kenya)	112	150 g	42	47
White, Type ▲, cooked in salted water, refrigerated 16–20h, reheated (India)	53	150 g	38	20
White, Type ▲, cooked 13 min, then baked 10 min (Italy)	104	150 g	30	31

Rye

FOOD	GI Value	Nominal Serving Size	Net Carb per Serving	GL per Serving
Whole kernels (Canada)	29	50 g (dry)	38	11
Whole kernels (average)	34	50 g (dry)	38	13

Tapioca

FOOD	GI Value	Nominal Serving Size	Net Carb per Serving	GL per Serving
Tapioca boiled with milk (General Mills, Canada)	81	250 g	18	14
Tapioca (Manihot utilissima) (India)	70	250 g	18	12

Wheat

FOOD	GI Value	Nominal Serving Size	Net Carb per Serving	GL per Serving
Cracked (bulgur), cooked (average)	48	150 g	26	12
Precooked kernels, durum, cooked 10 min (France)	50	50 g (dry)	33	17
Precooked kernels, durum, cooked 20 min (France)	52	50 g (dry)	37	19
Precooked kernels, in pouch, reheated (France)	40	125 g	39	16
Precooked kernels, quick-cooking (White Wings, Australia)	54	150 g	47	25

[0] indicates that the food has so little carbohydrate that the GI value cannot be tested. The GL, therefore, is 0. ▲ indicates brand not specified.

FOOD	GI Value	Nominal Serving Size	Net Carb per Serving	GL per Serving
Semolina, cooked (average)	55	150 g	11	6
Type ▲ (India)	90	50 g (dry)	38	34
Whole kernels (Canada)	42	50 g (dry)	33	14
Whole kernels (Canada)	48	50 g (dry)	33	16
Whole kernels (*Triticum aestivum*) (India)	30	50 g (dry)	38	11
Whole kernels, pressure cooked (Canada)	44	50 g (dry)	33	14
■ *average*	41	50 g (dry)	34	14

INFANT FORMULA AND BABY FOODS

[100 mL = 3.3 oz; 30 g = 1 oz]

Baby foods

FOOD	GI Value	Nominal Serving Size	Net Carb per Serving	GL per Serving
Apple, apricot, and banana, baby cereal	56	75 oz	13	7
Chicken and noodles with vegetables, strained	67	120 g	7	5
Sweetcorn and rice, baby	65	120 g	15	10
Creamed baby oatmeal	59	75 g	9	5
Farex™ baby rice (Heinz, Australia)	95	87 g	6	6
Rice pudding, baby	59	75 g	11	6

Infant formula

FOOD	GI Value	Nominal Serving Size	Net Carb per Serving	GL per Serving
Infasoy™, soy-based, milk-free (Wyeth, Australia)	55	100 mL	7	4
Karicare™ with omega oils (Nutricia, New Zealand)	35	100 mL	7	2
Nan-1™ with iron (Nestlé, Australia)	30	100 mL	8	2
S-26™ (Wyeth, Australia)	36	100 mL	7	3

[0] indicates that the food has so little carbohydrate that the GI value cannot be tested. The GL, therefore, is 0. ▲ indicates brand not specified.

FOOD	GI Value	Nominal Serving Size	Net Carb per Serving	GL per Serving

LEGUMES

[150 g = 5 oz]

Beans

FOOD	GI Value	Nominal Serving Size	Net Carb per Serving	GL per Serving
Baked, canned (average)	48	150 g	15	7
Black (*Phaseolus vulgaris* Linn), cooked (Philippines)	20	150 g	25	5
Butter (Canada)	36	150 g	20	7
Butter (South Africa)	28	150 g	20	5
Butter, dried, cooked (South Africa)	29	150 g	20	6
■ *average*	31	150 g	20	6
Butter, dried, cooked + 5 g sucrose (South Africa)	30	150 g	20	6
Butter, dried, cooked + 10 g sucrose (South Africa)	31	150 g	20	6
Butter, dried, cooked + 15 g sucrose (South Africa)	54	150 g	20	11
Dried, type ▲ (Italy)	36	150 g	30	11
Dried, type ▲ (Italy)	20	150 g	30	6
■ *average*	29	150 g	30	9
Kidney (Canada)	29	150 g	25	7
Kidney (Canada)	46	150 g	25	11
Kidney (*Phaseolus vulgaris* L.), red, cooked (Sweden)	25	150 g	25	6
Kidney (*Phaseolus vulgaris*) (India)	19	150 g	25	5
Kidney (USA)	23	150 g	25	6
Kidney, dried, cooked (Canada)	42	150 g	25	10
Kidney, dried, cooked (France)	23	150 g	25	6

[0] indicates that the food has so little carbohydrate that the GI value cannot be tested. The GL, therefore, is 0. ▲ indicates brand not specified.

FOOD	GI Value	Nominal Serving Size	Net Carb per Serving	GL per Serving
Kidney/white (*Phaseolus vulgaris* Linn), cooked (Philippines)	13	150 g	25	3
■ average	28	150 g	25	7
Kidney (*Phaseolus vulgaris* L.) autoclaved	34	150 g	25	8
Kidney, canned (Lancia-Bravo, Canada)	52	150 g	17	9
Kidney, soaked 12 h, stored moist 24 h, steamed 1 h (India)	70	150 g	25	17
Lima, baby, frozen (York, Canada)	32	150 g	30	10
Mung (*Phaseolus areus* Roxb), cooked (Philippines)	31	150 g	17	5
Mung, germinated (Australia)	25	150 g	17	4
Mung, pressure cooked (Australia)	42	150 g	17	7
Navy (King Grains, Canada)	39	150 g	30	12
Navy, cooked (Canada)	31	150 g	30	9
Navy, dried, cooked (Canada)	30	150 g	30	9
Navy, pressure cooked (King Grains, Canada)	29	150 g	33	9
Navy, pressure cooked (King Grains, Canada)	59	150 g	33	19
■ average	38	150 g	31	12
Pinto, canned in brine (Lancia-Bravo, Canada)	45	150 g	22	10
Pinto, cooked (Canada)	39	150 g	26	10
Romano (Canada)	46	150 g	18	8
Soy, canned (Canada)	14	150 g	6	1
Soy, cooked (Australia)	20	150 g	6	1
Soy, cooked (Canada)	15	150 g	6	1
■ average	18	150 g	6	1

[0] indicates that the food has so little carbohydrate that the GI value cannot be tested. The GL, therefore, is 0. ▲ indicates brand not specified.

FOOD	GI Value	Nominal Serving Size	Net Carb per Serving	GL per Serving
Lentils				
Green, dried, cooked (Australia)	37	150 g	14	5
Green, dried, cooked (Canada)	22	150 g	18	4
Green, dried, cooked (France)	30	150 g	18	6
■ *average*	30	150 g	17	5
Green, canned in brine (Lancia-Bravo Foods Ltd., Canada)	52	150 g	17	9
Red, dried, cooked (Canada)	18	150 g	18	3
Red, dried, cooked (Canada)	21	150 g	18	4
Red, dried, cooked (Canada)	31	150 g	18	6
Red, dried, cooked (Canada)	32	150 g	18	6
■ *average*	26	150 g	18	5
Type ▲ (average)	29	150 g	18	5
Peas				
Black-eyed (Canada)	50	150 g	21	11
Black-eyed (Canada)	33	150 g	21	7
■ *average*	42	150 g	21	9
Chickpeas/garbanzo beans (Canada)	35	150 g	24	8
Chickpeas/garbanzo beans (*Cicer arietinum* Linn), cooked (Philippines)	10	150 g	24	2
Chickpeas/garbanzo beans, dried, cooked (Canada)	31	150 g	24	7
■ *average*	25	150 g	24	6
Chickpeas/garbanzo beans, canned in brine (Lancia-Bravo, Canada)	42	150 g	22	9

[0] indicates that the food has so little carbohydrate that the GI value cannot be tested. The GL, therefore, is 0. ▲ indicates brand not specified.

FOOD	GI Value	Nominal Serving Size	Net Carb per Serving	GL per Serving
Chickpeas/garbanzo beans, curry, canned (Canasia, Canada)	41	150 g	16	7
Marrowfat, dried, cooked (average)	39	150 g	19	7
Split, yellow, cooked (Nupack, Canada)	32	150 g	19	6

MEAL-REPLACEMENT PRODUCTS

[250 mL = 8 oz; 30 g = 1 oz]

FOOD	GI Value	Nominal Serving Size	Net Carb per Serving	GL per Serving
Burn-it™ bar, chocolate deluxe	29	50 g	8	2
Burn-it™ bar, peanut butter	23	50 g	6	1
Designer chocolate, sugar-free, Worldwide Sport Nutrition low-carbohydrate products (USA)	14	35 g	22	3
Hazelnut and Apricot bar (Dietworks, Australia)	42	50 g	22	9
L.E.A.N Fibergy™ bar, Harvest Oat (Usana, USA▲)	45	50 g	29	13
Nutrimeal™, drink powder, Dutch Chocolate	26	250 mL	13	3
L.E.A.N (Life long) Nutribar™, Chocolate Crunch (Usana, USA)	32	40 g	19	6
L.E.A.N (Life long) Nutribar™, Peanut Crunch (Usana, USA)	30	40 g	19	6
■ average	31	40 g	19	6
Pure-protein™ bar, chewy choc-chip	30	80 g	14	4
Pure-protein™ bar, chocolate deluxe	38	80 g	13	5
Pure-protein™ bar, peanut butter	22	80 g	9	2
Pure-protein™ bar, strawberry shortcake	43	80 g	13	6
Pure-protein™ bar, white chocolate mousse	40	80 g	15	6
Pure-protein™ cookie, choc-chip cookie dough	25	55 g	11	3

[0] indicates that the food has so little carbohydrate that the GI value cannot be tested. The GL, therefore, is 0. ▲ indicates brand not specified.

FOOD	GI Value	Nominal Serving Size	Net Carb per Serving	GL per Serving
Pure-protein™ cookie, coconut	42	55 g	9	4
Pure-protein™ cookie, peanut butter	37	55 g	9	3
Ultra pure-protein™ shake, cappuccino	47	250 mL	1	1
Ultra pure-protein™ shake, frosty chocolate	37	250 mL	3	1
Ultra pure-protein™ shake, strawberry shortcake	42	250 mL	1	1
Ultra pure-protein™ shake, vanilla ice cream	32	250 mL	3	1

MIXED MEALS and CONVENIENCE FOODS

$$[\ 250 \text{ mL} = 8 \text{ oz}; 30 \text{ g} = 1 \text{ oz} \ ]$$

FOOD	GI Value	Nominal Serving Size	Net Carb per Serving	GL per Serving
Chicken nuggets, frozen, reheated (Australia)	46	100 g	16	7
Fish fillet, reduced fat, breaded (Maggi)	43	85 g	16	7
Fish fingers (Canada)	38	100 g	19	7
Greek lentil stew with a bread roll, homemade (Australia)	40	360 g	37	15
Kugel (Polish dish containing egg noodles, sugar, cheese, and raisins) (Israel)	65	150 g	48	31
Lean Cuisine™, chicken with rice (Nestlé, Australia)	36	400 g	68	24
Macaroni and cheese, boxed (Kraft, Canada)	64	180 g	51	32
Pies, beef, party size (Farmland, Australia)	45	100 g	27	12
Pizza, cheese (Pillsbury, Canada)	60	100 g	27	16
Pizza, plain (Italy)	80	100 g	27	22
Pizza, Super Supreme, pan (Pizza Hut, Australia)	36	100 g	24	9
Pizza, Super Supreme, thin and crispy (Pizza Hut, Australia)	30	100 g	22	7

[0] indicates that the food has so little carbohydrate that the GI value cannot be tested. The GL, therefore, is 0. ▲ indicates brand not specified.

FOOD	GI Value	Nominal Serving Size	Net Carb per Serving	GL per Serving
Pizza, Vegetarian Supreme, thin and crispy (Pizza Hut, Australia)	49	100 g	25	12
Sausage, Type ▲ (Canada)	28	100 g	3	1
Sirloin chop with mixed vegetables and mashed potato (Australia)	66	360 g	53	35
Spaghetti bolognese, homemade (Australia)	52	360 g	48	25
Spaghetti, gluten-free, canned in tomato sauce (Orgran, Australia)	68	220 g	27	19
Stir-fried vegetables with chicken and rice, homemade (Australia)	73	360 g	75	55
Sushi, roasted sea algae, vinegar, and rice (Japan)	55	100 g	37	20
Sushi, salmon (Australia)	48	100 g	36	17
■ average	52	100 g	37	19
Taco shells, cornmeal-based, baked (Old El Paso, Canada)	68	20 g	12	8
Tortellini, cheese (Stouffer, Canada)	50	180 g	21	10
Tuna patty, reduced fat	45	84 g	17	80
White boiled rice, grilled beefburger, cheese and butter (France)	22	440 g	50	14
White boiled rice, grilled beefburger, cheese and butter (France)	22	440 g	50	11
■ average	25	440 g	50	13
White bread with butter (Canada)	59	100 g	48	29
White bread with butter and skim-milk cheese (Canada)	62	100 g	38	23
White bread with skim-milk cheese (Canada)	55	100 g	47	26

[0] indicates that the food has so little carbohydrate that the GI value cannot be tested. The GL, therefore, is 0. ▲ indicates brand not specified.

FOOD	GI Value	Nominal Serving Size	Net Carb per Serving	GL per Serving
White bread, butter, regular cow's milk, cheese, and fresh cucumber (Sweden)	55	200 g	68	38
White bread, butter, yogurt, and pickled cucumber (Sweden)	39	200 g	28	11
White/whole-wheat bread with peanut butter (Canada)	51	100 g	44	23
White/whole-wheat bread with peanut butter (Canada)	67	100 g	44	30
■ average	59	100 g	44	26

NOODLES

[180 g = 6 oz]

FOOD	GI Value	Nominal Serving Size	Net Carb per Serving	GL per Serving
Instant, average	47	180 g	40	19
Lungkow beanthread (National Cereals, China)	26	180 g	45	12
Longkou beanthread (Yantai, China)	39	180 g	45	18
Rice, dried, cooked (Thai World, Thailand)	61	180 g	39	23
Rice, freshly made, cooked (Sydney, Australia)	40	180 g	39	15
Udon, plain, reheated 5 min (Australia)	62	180 g	48	30

PASTA

[180 g = 6 oz]

FOOD	GI Value	Nominal Serving Size	Net Carb per Serving	GL per Serving
Capellini (Primo, Canada)	45	180 g	45	20
Corn, gluten-free (Orgran, Australia)	78	180 g	42	32
Fettuccine, egg	32	180 g	46	15
Fettuccine, egg (Mother Earth, Australia)	47	180 g	46	22
■ average	40	180 g	46	18

[0] indicates that the food has so little carbohydrate that the GI value cannot be tested. The GL, therefore, is 0. ▲ indicates brand not specified.

FOOD	GI Value	Nominal Serving Size	Net Carb per Serving	GI per Serving
Gluten free pasta, maize starch, cooked (UK)	54	180 g	42	22
Gnocchi, ▲ (Latina, Australia)	68	180 g	48	33
Linguine, thick, durum wheat, white, fresh (Sweden)	43	180 g	48	21
Linguine, thick, fresh, durum wheat flour (Sweden)	48	180 g	48	23
■ average	46	180 g	48	22
Linguine, thin, durum wheat (Sweden)	49	180 g	48	23
Linguine, thin, fresh, durum wheat flour (Sweden)	61	180 g	48	29
■ average	52	180 g	45	23
Macaroni, plain, cooked (Turkey)	48	180 g	49	23
Macaroni, plain, cooked 5 min (Lancia-Bravo, Canada)	45	180 g	49	22
■ average	47	180 g	48	23
Ravioli (Australia)	39	180 g	38	15
Rice and maize, gluten-free, Ris'O'Mais (Orgran, Australia)	76	180 g	49	37
Rice, brown, cooked 16 min (Rice Growers, Australia)	92	180 g	38	35
Rice, vermicelli, Kongmoon (China)	58	180 g	39	22
Spaghetti, cooked 5 min (Canada)	37	180 g	48	18
Spaghetti, cooked 5 min (Lancia-Bravo, Canada)	32	180 g	48	15
Spaghetti, cooked 5 min (Middle East)	44	180 g	48	21
■ average	38	180 g	48	18

[0] indicates that the food has so little carbohydrate that the GI value cannot be tested. The GL, therefore, is 0. ▲ indicates brand not specified.

FOOD	GI Value	Nominal Serving Size	Net Carb per Serving	GL per Serving
Spaghetti, cooked 11 min	59	180 g	48	28
Spaghetti, cooked 16.5 min	65	180 g	48	31
Spaghetti, cooked 22 min	46	180 g	48	22
▪ average	57	180 g	48	27
Spaghetti, protein enriched, cooked 7 min (Catelli, Canada)	27	180 g	52	14
Spaghetti, white, cooked 15 min (Canada)	41	180 g	48	20
Spaghetti, white, cooked 15 min (Lancia-Bravo, Canada)	32	180 g	48	15
Spaghetti, white, durum wheat flour, cooked 12 min (Starhushålls, Sweden)	47	180 g	48	23
Spaghetti, white, durum wheat, cooked 10 min (Barilla, Italy)	58	180 g	48	28
Spaghetti, white, durum wheat flour, cooked 12 min (Sweden)	53	180 g	48	25
Spaghetti, white, cooked 15 min in salted water (Unico, Canada)	44	180 g	48	21
▪ average	44	180 g	48	21
Spaghetti, durum wheat, cooked 20 min (USA)	64	180 g	43	27
Spaghetti, white, durum wheat, cooked 20 min (Australia)	58	180 g	44	26
▪ average	61	180 g	44	27
Spaghetti, white (Australia)	38	180 g	44	17
Spaghetti, white (Canada)	47	180 g	48	23
Spaghetti, white (Denmark)	33	180 g	48	16
Spaghetti, white (Vetta, Australia)	49	180 g	44	22

[0] indicates that the food has so little carbohydrate that the GI value cannot be tested. The GL, therefore, is 0. ▲ indicates brand not specified.

FOOD	GI Value	Nominal Serving Size	Net Carb per Serving	GL per Serving
Spaghetti, white, durum wheat (Catelli, Canada)	34	180 g	48	16
■ *average*	42	180 g	47	20
Spaghetti, whole wheat (Canada)	42	180 g	40	17
Spaghetti, whole wheat (USA)	32	180 g	44	14
■ *average*	37	180 g	42	16
Spirali, durum wheat, white, cooked (Vetta, Australia)	43	180 g	44	19
Star pastina, white, cooked 5 minutes (Lancia-Bravo, Canada)	38	180 g	48	18
Vermicelli, white, cooked (Australia)	35	180 g	44	16

PROTEIN FOODS

[120 g = 4 oz]

FOOD	GI Value	Nominal Serving Size	Net Carb per Serving	GL per Serving
Beef	[0]	120 g	0	0
Cheese	[0]	120 g	0	0
Cold cuts	[0]	120 g	0	0
Eggs	[0]	120 g	0	0
Fish	[0]	120 g	0	0
Lamb	[0]	120 g	0	0
Pork	[0]	120 g	0	0
Shellfish (shrimp, crab, lobster, etc.)	[0]	120 g	0	0
Veal	[0]	120 g	0	0

SNACK FOODS AND CANDY

[30 g = 1 oz]

Burger rings

FOOD	GI Value	Nominal Serving Size	Net Carb per Serving	GL per Serving
Burger Rings™ (Smith's, Australia)	90	50 g	31	28

[0] indicates that the food has so little carbohydrate that the GI value cannot be tested. The GL, therefore, is 0. ▲ indicates brand not specified.

FOOD	GI Value	Nominal Serving Size	Net Carb per Serving	GL per Serving
Candy				
Jelly beans, assorted colors (average)	78	30 g	28	22
Life Savers®, peppermint candy (Nestlé, Australia)	70	30 g	30	21
Nougat, Jijona (La Fama, Spain)	32	30 g	12	4
Skittles® (Australia)	70	50 g	45	32
Sunripe school straps	40	15 g	11	4
Chips				
Cheese Twisties™ (Smith's, Australia)	74	50 g	29	22
Corn, plain, salted (Doritos™, Australia)	42	50 g	25	11
Corn, Nachips™ (Old El Paso, Canada)	74	50 g	29	21
■ average	63	50 g	26	17
Crisps, potato, plain, salted (Arnotts, Australia)	57	50 g	18	10
Crisps, potato, plain, salted (Canada)	51	50 g	24	12
■ average	54	50 g	21	11
Chocolate bars				
Milk, with sucrose (Belgium)	34	50 g	22	7
Milk (Cadbury's, Australia)	49	50 g	30	14
Milk, Dove® (Mars, Australia)	45	50 g	30	13
Milk (Nestlé, Australia)	42	50 g	31	13
■ average	43	50 g	28	12
Milk, plain, low-sugar with maltitol (Belgium)	35	50 g	22	8
Mars Bar® (Australia)	62	60 g	40	25
Mars Bar® (USA)	68	60 g	40	27
■ average	65	60 g	40	26

[0] indicates that the food has so little carbohydrate that the GI value cannot be tested. The GL, therefore, is 0. ▲ indicates brand not specified.

FOOD	GI Value	Nominal Serving Size	Net Carb per Serving	GL per Serving
Snickers Bar® (Australia)	41	60 g	36	15
Snickers Bar® (USA)	68	60 g	34	23
■ average	55	60 g	35	19
White, Milky Bar® (Nestlé, Australia)	44	50 g	29	13

Chocolate candy

FOOD	GI Value	Nominal Serving Size	Net Carb per Serving	GL per Serving
M & M's®, peanut (Australia)	33	30 g	17	6

Chocolate spread

FOOD	GI Value	Nominal Serving Size	Net Carb per Serving	GL per Serving
Nutella®, chocolate hazelnut spread (Australia)	33	20 g	12	4

Dried-fruit bars and snacks

FOOD	GI Value	Nominal Serving Size	Net Carb per Serving	GL per Serving
Apricot-filled fruit bar (Mother Earth, New Zealand)	50	50 g	34	17
Fruity Bitz™, apricot (Blackmores, Australia)	42	15 g	12	5
Fruity Bitz™, berry (Blackmores, Australia)	35	15 g	12	4
Fruity Bitz™, tropical (Blackmores, Australia)	41	15 g	11	5
■ average	39	15 g	12	4
Heinz Kidz™ Fruit Fingers, banana (Heinz, Australia)	61	30 g	20	12
Real Fruit Bars, strawberry (Uncle Toby's, Australia)	90	30 g	26	23
Roll-Ups® (Uncle Toby's, Australia)	99	30 g	25	24

Nuts

FOOD	GI Value	Nominal Serving Size	Net Carb per Serving	GL per Serving
Cashews, salted (Coles Supermarkets, Australia)	22	50 g	13	3

[0] indicates that the food has so little carbohydrate that the GI value cannot be tested. The GL, therefore, is 0. ▲ indicates brand not specified.

FOOD	GI Value	Nominal Serving Size	Net Carb per Serving	GL per Serving
Peanuts, crushed (South Africa)	7	50 g	4	0
Peanuts (Canada)	13	50 g	7	1
Peanuts (Mexico)	23	50 g	7	2
■ average	14	50 g	6	1
Pecans	[0]	50 g	0	0
Popcorn				
Plain, cooked in microwave oven (Green's, Australia)	55	20 g	11	6
Plain, cooked in microwave oven (Uncle Toby's, Australia)	89	20 g	11	10
■ average	72	20 g	11	8
Pop Tarts™				
Double choc (Kellogg's, Australia)	70	50 g	35	24
Pretzels				
Parker's, Australia	83	30 g	20	16
Snack bars				
Apple Cinnamon (Con Agra, USA)	40	50 g	29	12
Kudos Whole Grain Bars, chocolate chip (USA)	62	50 g	32	20
Muesli bar containing dried fruit (Uncle Toby's, Australia)	61	30 g	21	13
Peanut Butter & Choc-Chip (USA)	37	50 g	27	10
Twix® Cookie Bar, caramel (USA)	44	60 g	39	17
Sports bars				
Ironman PR bar®, chocolate (USA)	39	65 g	26	10
PowerBar®, chocolate (average)	56	65 g	42	24

[0] indicates that the food has so little carbohydrate that the GI value cannot be tested. The GL, therefore, is 0. ▲ indicates brand not specified.

FOOD	GI Value	Nominal Serving Size	Net Carb per Serving	GL per Serving

SOUPS

[250 g = 8 oz (approx.)]

FOOD	GI Value	Nominal Serving Size	Net Carb per Serving	GL per Serving
Black Bean (Wil-Pack, USA)	64	250 g	27	17
Green Pea, canned (Campbell's, Canada)	66	250 g	41	27
Lentil, canned (Unico, Canada)	44	250 g	21	9
Minestrone, Country Ladle™ (Campbell's, Australia)	39	250 g	18	7
Noodle soup (Turkish soup with stock and noodles)	1	250 g	9	0
Split Pea (Wil-Pak, USA)	60	250 g	27	16
Tomato soup (Canada)	38	250 g	17	6

SPECIAL DIETARY PRODUCTS

[240 mL = 8 oz; 30 g = 1 oz]

FOOD	GI Value	Nominal Serving Size	Net Carb per Serving	GL per Serving
Choice DM™, vanilla (Mead Johnson, USA)	23	237 mL	24	6
Enercal Plus™ (Wyeth-Ayerst, USA)	61	237 mL	40	24
Enrich Plus shake, vanilla (Ross, USA)	58	200 mL	40	23
Ensure™ (Abbott, Australia)	50	237 mL	40	19
Ensure™, vanilla (Abbott, Australia)	48	250 mL	34	16
Ensure™ bar, chocolate fudge brownie (Abbott, Australia)	43	38 g	20	8
Ensure Plus™, vanilla (Abbott, Australia)	40	237 mL	47	19
Ensure Pudding™, vanilla (Abbott, USA)	36	113 g	26	9
Glucerna™, vanilla (Abbott, USA)	31	237 g	23	7
Glucerna™ bar, lemon crunch (Abbott, USA)	27	38 g	20	5
Glucerna™ SR shake, vanilla (Abbott, USA)	19	230 mL	24	5
Jevity™ (Abbott, Australia)	48	237 mL	36	17

[0] indicates that the food has so little carbohydrate that the GI value cannot be tested. The GL, therefore, is 0. ▲ indicates brand not specified.

FOOD	GI Value	Nominal Serving Size	Net Carb per Serving	GL per Serving
Resource Diabetic™, vanilla (Novartis, USA)	34	237 mL	23	8
Resource Diabetic™, chocolate (Novartis, New Zealand)	16	237 mL	41	7
Resource™ thickened orange juice (Novartis, New Zealand)	47	237 mL	39	18
Resource™ thickened orange juice (Novartis, New Zealand)	54	237 mL	36	19
Resource™ fruit beverage, peach flavor (Novartis, New Zealand)	40	237 mL	41	16
Resource Plus, chocolate (Novartis, New Zealand)	43	237 mL	52	22
Sustagen™, Dutch Chocolate (Mead Johnson, Australia)	31	250 mL	41	13
Sustagen™ Hospital with extra fiber (Mead Johnson, Australia)	33	250 mL	44	15
Sustagen™ Instant Pudding, vanilla (Mead Johnson, Australia)	27	250 g	47	13
Ultracal™ with fiber (Mead Johnson, USA)	40	237 mL	29	12

SUGARS

[10 g = 2½ tsp = 0.3 oz; 25 g = ½ Tbsp = 0.8 oz]

FOOD	GI Value	Nominal Serving Size	Net Carb per Serving	GL per Serving
Blue Agave, Organic Agave Cactus Nectar, light, (Western Commerce, USA) 90% fructose	11	10 g	8	1
Blue Agave, Organic Agave Cactus Nectar, light, 97% fructose (Western Commerce, USA)	10	10 g	8	1
Fructose	19	10 g	10	2
Glucose	100	10 g	10	10
Glucose, consumed with 3 grams American ginseng	78	10 g	10	8
Glucose, consumed with gum/fiber, 14.5 g guar gum	62	10 g	10	6

[0] indicates that the food has so little carbohydrate that the GI value cannot be tested. The GL, therefore, is 0. ▲ indicates brand not specified.

FOOD	GI Value	Nominal Serving Size	Net Carb per Serving	GI per Serving
Glucose, consumed with gum/fiber, 14.5 g oat gum (78% oat ß-glucan)	57	10 g	10	6
Glucose, consumed with gum/fiber, 15 g apple and orange fiber (FITA, Australia)	79	10 g	8	6
Glucose, consumed with gum/fiber, 20 g acacia gum	85	10 g	10	9
Honey, Commercial Blend (Australia)	62	25 g	18	11
Honey, Commercial Blend (Australia)	72	25 g	13	9
Honey, Iron Bark (Australia)	48	25 g	15	7
Honey, Locust (Romania)	32	25 g	21	7
Honey, pure (Capilano, Australia)	58	25 g	21	12
Honey, Red Gum (Australia)	46	25 g	18	8
Honey, Salvation Jane (Australia)	64	25 g	15	10
Honey, Stringy Bark (Australia)	44	25 g	21	9
Honey, Yapunya (Australia)	52	25 g	17	9
Honey, Yellow box (Australia)	35	25 g	18	6
Honey ▲ (Canada)	87	25 g	21	18
■ *average*	55	25 g	18	10
Lactose	46	10 g	10	5
Maltose	105	10 g	10	11
Sucrose	61	10 g	10	6

VEGETABLES

	[80 g = 2.7 oz; 150 g = 5 oz]			
Artichokes	[0]	80 g	0	0
Avocado	[0]	80 g	0	0
Beet (Canada)	64	80 g	7	5
Bok choy, raw	[0]	80 g	0	0
Broad beans (Canada)	79	80 g	11	9

[0] indicates that the food has so little carbohydrate that the GI value cannot be tested. The GL, therefore, is 0. ▲ indicates brand not specified.

FOOD	GI Value	Nominal Serving Size	Net Carb per Serving	GL per Serving
Broccoli, raw	[0]	80 g	0	0
Cabbage, raw	[0]	80 g	0	0
Carrots, peeled, cooked (Australia)	49	80 g	5	2
Cassava, cooked, with salt (Kenya, Africa)	46	100 g	27	12
Cauliflower	[0]	80 g	0	0
Celery	[0]	80 g	0	0
Corn, sweet (Canada)	59	80 g	18	11
Corn, sweet (South Africa)	62	80 g	18	11
Corn, sweet, cooked (USA)	60	80 g	18	11
Corn, sweet, "Honey & Pearl" variety (New Zealand)	37	80 g	16	6
Corn, sweet, on the cob, cooked (Australia)	48	80 g	16	8
■ average	54	80 g	17	9
Corn, sweet, diet-pack (USA)	46	80 g	14	7
Corn, sweet, frozen (Canada)	47	80 g	15	7
Cucumber	[0]	80 g	0	0
French beans (runner beans), cooked	[0]	80 g	0	0
Leafy vegetables (spinach, arugula, etc.), raw	[0]	80 g	0	0
Lettuce	[0]	80 g	0	0
Parsnips	97	80 g	12	12
Peas, frozen, cooked (Canada)	39	80 g	7	3
Peas, frozen, cooked (Canada)	51	80 g	7	4
■ average	48	80 g	7	3
Pepper	[0]	80 g	0	0
Potato dumplings (Italy)	52	150 g	45	24

[0] indicates that the food has so little carbohydrate that the GI value cannot be tested. The GL, therefore, is 0. ▲ indicates brand not specified.

FOOD	GI Value	Nominal Serving Size	Net Carb per Serving	GL per Serving
Potato, boiled, Desiree (Australia)	101	150 g	17	17
Potato, boiled, Nardine (New Zealand)	70	150 g	25	18
Potato, boiled, Ontario (Canada)	58	150 g	27	16
Potato, boiled, Pontiac (Australia)	88	150 g	18	16
Potato, boiled, Prince Edward Island (Canada)	63	150 g	18	11
Potato, boiled, Sebago (Australia)	87	150 g	17	14
Potato, boiled, Type NS ▲ (India)	76	150 g	34	26
Potato, boiled, Type NS ▲ refrigerated, reheated (India)	23	150 g	34	8
Potato, boiled, white (Canada)	54	150 g	27	15
Potato, boiled, white (Romania)	41	150 g	30	12
Potato, russet, baked without fat (average)	85	150 g	30	26
Potato, white, Ontario, baked in skin (Canada)	60	150 g	30	18
Potato, canned, Prince Edward Island (Cobi Foods, Canada)	61	150 g	18	11
Potato, canned, new (Edgell's, Australia)	65	150 g	18	12
■ *average*	63	150 g	18	11
Potato, French fries, frozen and reheated (Cavendish Farms, Canada)	75	150 g	29	22
Potato, instant (average)	85	150 g	20	17
Potato, mashed, Prince Edward Island (Canada)	73	150 g	18	13
Potato, Pontiac (Australia)	91	150 g	20	18
■ *average*	92	150 g	20	18
Potato, microwaved, Pontiac, peeled, cooked on high for 6–7.5 min (Australia)	79	150 g	18	14

[0] indicates that the food has so little carbohydrate that the GI value cannot be tested. The GL, therefore, is 0. ▲ indicates brand not specified.

FOOD	GI Value	Nominal Serving Size	Net Carb per Serving	GL per Serving
Potato, microwaved, Type NS ▲ (USA)	82	150 g	33	27
Potato, new (average)	62	150 g	21	13
Potato, steamed, peeled (India)	65	150 g	27	18
Potato, sweet, Ipomoea batatas (Australia)	44	150 g	25	11
Potato, sweet, Type NSs (Canada)	48	150 g	34	16
Potato, sweet (Canada)	59	150 g	30	18
Potato, sweet, kumara (New Zealand)	78	150 g	25	20
■ *average*	61	150 g	28	17
Pumpkin (South Africa)	75	80 g	4	3
Rutabaga (Canada)	72	150 g	10	7
Squash, raw	[0]	80 g	0	0
Taro (average)	55	150 g	8	4
Yam (average)	37	150 g	36	13

[0] indicates that the food has so little carbohydrate that the GI value cannot be tested. The GL, therefore, is 0. ▲ indicates brand not specified.

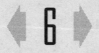

LOW TO HIGH GI VALUES

*F*OR THOSE WHO wish to choose a diet with the low-est GI values possible, we've created the following listing in order of GI values (i.e., from lowest to highest value). We've also divided the list into food categories, so that when you want to find a low-GI vegetable or fruit, for example, the information is at your fingertips. The categories are:

- bakery products
- beverages
- breads
- breakfast foods
- cookies
- crackers
- dairy products and alternatives
- fruits and fruit products
- grains
- infant formulas and baby foods

- legumes
- meal-replacement products
- mixed meals and convenience foods
- noodles
- pasta
- protein foods
- snack foods and candy
- soups
- special dietary products
- sugars
- vegetables

As we discuss in *The New Glucose Revolution,* it's not necessary to eat all of your carbohydrates from low-GI sources. If half of your carbohydrate choices have low-GI values, you're doing well. If you also eat a low-GI food at each meal, you'll be reducing the GI values overall.

FOOD	LOW	INTERMEDIATE	HIGH

BAKERY PRODUCTS

Cakes

FOOD	LOW	INTERMEDIATE	HIGH
Banana	○		
Chocolate, with chocolate frosting	○		
Pound	○		
Sponge	○		
Vanilla	○		
Angel food		◑	
Flan		◑	

Muffins

FOOD	LOW	INTERMEDIATE	HIGH
Apple with sugar or artificial sweeteners	○		
Apple, oat, and raisin	○		
Banana, oat and honey		◑	
Bran		◑	
Blueberry		◑	
Carrot		◑	
Oatmeal, made from mix, Quaker Oats		◑	
Cupcake, iced			●
Scone, plain			●

Pastries

FOOD	LOW	INTERMEDIATE	HIGH
Croissant		◑	
Doughnut, cake-type			●

BEVERAGES

Alcoholic

FOOD	LOW	INTERMEDIATE	HIGH
Beer	○		
Brandy	○		

FOOD	LOW	INTERMEDIATE	HIGH
Gin	○		
Sherry	○		
Whiskey	○		
Wine, red	○		
Wine, white	○		
Juices			
Apple, with sugar or artificial sweetener	○		
Carrot, fresh	○		
Grapefruit, unsweetened	○		
Pineapple, unsweetened	○		
Tomato, canned, no added sugar	○		
Smoothies and Shakes			
Raspberry	○		
Soy	○		
Soft Drinks			
Coke		◑	
Fanta®		◑	
Sports drinks			
Gatorade®			●

BREADS

Fruit			
Muesli, made from mix	○		
Happiness™, cinnamon, raisin, pecan		◑	
Gluten-free			
Fiber-enriched			●
White			●

FOOD	LOW	INTERMEDIATE	HIGH
Rye			
Pumpernickel	○		
Sourdough	○		
Cocktail		◑	
Light		◑	
Whole-wheat		◑	
Spelt			
Multigrain	○		
White			
Wheat			
100% Whole Grain	○		
Soy & Linseed bread machine mix	○		
Flatbread, Indian		◑	
Hearty 7 Grain		◑	
Pita, plain		◑	
Bagel			
Baguette			●
Bread stuffing			
English Muffin™			
Flatbread, Middle Eastern			
Italian			
Lebanese, white			●
White, enriched			
Whole-wheat			

FOOD	LOW	INTERMEDIATE	HIGH

BREAKFAST FOODS

Breakfast cereal bars

Rice Krispies Treat		◐	

Cooked cereals

Hot cereal, apple & cinnamon, Con Agra	○		
Old-fashioned oats	○		
Cream of Wheat™, regular, Nabisco		◐	
One Minute Oats, Quaker Oats		◐	
Quick Oats, Quaker Oats		◐	
Cream of Wheat™, instant, Nabisco			●
Oatmeal, instant			●

Grain products

Pancakes, prepared from mix	○		
Pancakes, buckwheat, gluten-free, made from mix			●
Waffles, Aunt Jemima®			●

Ready-to-eat cereals

All-Bran®, Kellogg's	○		
Complete™ Bran Flakes, Kellogg's	○		
Bran Buds™, Kellogg's		◐	
Bran Chex™, Kellogg's		◐	
Froot Loops™, Kellogg's		◐	
Frosted Flakes™, Kellogg's		◐	
Just Right™, Kellogg's		◐	
Life™, Quaker Oats		◐	
Nutrigrain™, Kellogg's		◐	
Oat bran, raw, Quaker Oats		◐	
Puffed Wheat, Quaker Oats		◐	

FOOD	LOW	INTERMEDIATE	HIGH
Raisin Bran™, Kellogg's		◑	
Special K™, Kellogg's		◑	
Bran Flakes™, Kellogg's			●
Cheerios™, General Mills			●
Corn Chex™, Kellogg's			●
Corn Flakes™, Kellogg's			●
Corn Pops™, Kellogg's			●
Grapenuts™, Post			●
Rice Krispies™, Kellogg's			●
Shredded Wheat™, Nabisco			●
Team™ Flakes, Nabisco			●
Total™			●
Weetabix™			●

COOKIES

FOOD	LOW	INTERMEDIATE	HIGH
Hearty Oatmeal, Fifty-50	○		
Oatmeal, Sugar-Free, Fifty-50	○		
Vanilla wafers, creme filled, Fifty-50	○		
Arrowroot		◑	
Digestives		◑	
Tea biscuits		◑	
Shortbread		◑	
Vanilla wafers			●

CRACKERS

FOOD	LOW	INTERMEDIATE	HIGH
Breton wheat		◑	
Melba Toast		◑	
Rye crispbread		◑	
Ryvita™		◑	
Stoned Wheat Thins		◑	
Water		◑	

FOOD	LOW	INTERMEDIATE	HIGH
Kavli™ Norwegian Crispbread			●
Premium soda (Saltines)			●
Rice cakes, puffed			●

DAIRY PRODUCTS AND ALTERNATIVES

Custard

Homemade	○		

Ice cream

Regular	○		

Milk

Low-fat, chocolate, with aspartame	○		
Low-fat, chocolate, with sugar	○		
Skim	○		
Whole	○		
Condensed, sweetened			●

Mousse

Butterscotch, low-fat, Nestlé	○		
Chocolate, low-fat, Nestlé	○		
French vanilla, low-fat, Nestlé	○		
Hazelnut, low-fat, Nestlé	○		
Mango, low-fat, Nestlé	○		
Mixed berry, low-fat, Nestlé	○		
Strawberry, low-fat, Nestlé	○		

Pudding

Instant, chocolate, made with milk	○		
Instant, vanilla, made with milk	○		

FOOD	LOW	INTERMEDIATE	HIGH
Soy milk			
Reduced fat	○		
Whole	○		
Soy yogurt			
Tofu-based frozen dessert, chocolate			●
Yogurt			
Low-fat, fruit, with aspartame	○		
Low-fat, fruit, with sugar	○		
Nonfat, French vanilla, with sugar	○		
Nonfat, strawberry, with sugar	○		

FRUIT and FRUIT PRODUCTS

FOOD	LOW	INTERMEDIATE	HIGH
Apple, fresh	○		
Apricot, fresh	○		
Banana, fresh	○		
Cantaloupe, fresh	○		
Cherries, fresh	○		
Grapefruit, fresh	○		
Grapes, fresh	○		
Kiwi, fresh	○		
Mango, fresh	○		
Orange, fresh	○		
Peach, canned in natural juice	○		
Peach, fresh	○		
Pear, canned in pear juice	○		
Pear, fresh	○		
Plum, fresh	○		
Prunes, pitted	○		
Strawberries, fresh	○		
Strawberry jam	○		
Figs, dried		◑	

FOOD	LOW	INTERMEDIATE	HIGH
Fruit cocktail, canned		◑	
Papaya, fresh		◑	
Peach, canned in heavy syrup		◑	
Peach, canned in light syrup		◑	
Pineapple, fresh		◑	
Raisins/sultanas		◑	
Dates, dried			●
Lychee, canned in syrup, drained			●
Watermelon, fresh			●

GRAINS

FOOD	LOW	INTERMEDIATE	HIGH
Barley, cracked	○		
Barley, pearled	○		
Buckwheat	○		
Buckwheat groats	○		
Bulgur	○		
Corn, canned, no salt added	○		
Rice, brown	○		
Rice, Cajun Style, Uncle Ben's®	○		
Rice, Long Grain and Wild, Uncle Ben's®	○		
Rice, parboiled, converted, white, cooked 20–30 min, Uncle Ben's®	○		
Barley, rolled		◑	
Corn, fresh		◑	
Cornmeal		◑	
Couscous		◑	
Rice, arborio (risotto)		◑	
Rice, Basmati		◑	
Rice, Garden Style, Uncle Ben's®		◑	
Rice, parboiled, long grain, cooked 10 minutes		◑	
Millet			●

FOOD	LOW	INTERMEDIATE	HIGH
Rice, sticky			●
Rice, parboiled			●
Tapioca boiled with milk			●

INFANT FORMULA AND BABY FOODS

Baby foods

Apple, apricot, and banana, baby cereal		◐	
Chicken and noodles with vegetables, strained		◐	
Corn and rice, baby		◐	
Oatmeal, creamed, baby		◐	
Rice pudding, baby		◐	

Infant formula

SMA, 20 cal./fl oz, Wyeth	○		
Nursoy, soy-based, milk-free, Wyeth		◐	

LEGUMES

Beans

Baked, canned	○		
Butter, dried and cooked	○		
Kidney, canned	○		
Lima, baby, frozen	○		
Mung, cooked	○		
Navy, dried and cooked	○		
Pinto, cooked	○		
Soy, canned	○		

Lentils

Green, dried and cooked	○		
Red, dried and cooked	○		

FOOD	LOW	INTERMEDIATE	HIGH
Peas			
Black-eyed	○		
Chickpeas/garbanzo beans, canned	○		
Split, yellow, cooked	○		

MEAL-REPLACEMENT PRODUCTS

FOOD	LOW	INTERMEDIATE	HIGH
Designer chocolate, sugar-free, Worldwide Sport Nutrition low-carbohydrate products	○		
L.E.A.N Fibergy™ bar, Harvest Oat, Usana	○		
L.E.A.N (Life long) Nutribar™, Peanut Crunch, Usana	○		
L.E.A.N (Life long) Nutribar™, Chocolate Crunch, Usana	○		

MIXED MEALS AND CONVENIENCE FOODS

FOOD	LOW	INTERMEDIATE	HIGH
Chicken nuggets, frozen, reheated	○		
Fish fillet, reduced fat, breaded	○		
Fish sticks	○		
Greek lentil stew with a bread roll, homemade	○		
Lean Cuisine™, chicken with rice	○		
Pizza, Super Supreme, pan, Pizza Hut	○		
Pizza, Super Supreme, thin and crispy, Pizza Hut	○		
Pizza, Vegetarian Supreme, thin and crispy, Pizza Hut	○		
Spaghetti Bolognese	○		
Sushi, salmon	○		
Tortellini, cheese, Stouffer	○		
Tuna patty, reduced fat	○		
Cheese sandwich, white bread		◑	
Kugel		◑	
Macaroni and cheese, boxed, Kraft		◑	
Peanut-butter sandwich, white/whole-wheat bread		◑	
Pizza, cheese, Pillsbury		◑	

food	LOW	INTERMEDIATE	HIGH
Spaghetti, gluten-free, canned in tomato sauce		◑	
Sushi, roasted sea algae, vinegar and rice		◑	
Taco shells, cornmeal-based, baked, El Paso		◑	
White bread and butter		◑	
Stir-fried vegetables with chicken and rice, homemade			●

NOODLES

Instant	○		
Mung bean, Lungkow beanthread	○		
Rice, fresh, cooked	○		
Rice, dried, cooked		◑	
Udon, plain, reheated 5 min		◑	

PAƷTA

Capellini	○		
Fettuccine, egg	○		
Gluten-free, cornstarch	○		
Linguine, thick, fresh, durum wheat, white	○		
Linguine, thin, fresh, durum wheat	○		
Macaroni, plain, cooked	○		
Ravioli	○		
Spaghetti, cooked 5 min	○		
Spaghetti, cooked 22 min	○		
Spaghetti, protein enriched, cooked 7 min	○		
Spaghetti, whole wheat	○		
Spirali, cooked, durum wheat	○		
Star pastina, cooked 5 min	○		
Tortellini	○		
Vermicelli	○		
Gnocchi		◑	

FOOD	LOW	INTERMEDIATE	HIGH
Rice vermicelli		◑	
Spaghetti, cooked 10 min, Barilla		◑	
Corn, gluten-free			●
Rice and corn, gluten-free			●
Rice, brown, cooked 16 min			●

PROTEIN FOODS

FOOD	LOW	INTERMEDIATE	HIGH
Beef	○		
Cheese	○		
Cold cuts	○		
Eggs	○		
Fish	○		
Lamb	○		
Pork	○		
Sausages	○		
Shellfish (shrimp, crab, lobster, etc.)	○		
Veal	○		

SNACK FOODS AND CANDY

Candy

FOOD	LOW	INTERMEDIATE	HIGH
Nougat	○		
Jelly beans			●
Life Savers®			●
Skittles®			●

Chips

FOOD	LOW	INTERMEDIATE	HIGH
Corn, plain, salted, Doritos™	○		
Potato, plain, salted	○		

Chocolate bars

FOOD	LOW	INTERMEDIATE	HIGH
Milk, Cadbury's	○		

FOOD	LOW	INTERMEDIATE	HIGH
Milk, Dove®, Mars	○		
Milk, Nestlé	○		
White, Milky Bar®	○		
Mars Bar®		◑	
Snickers Bar®		◑	

Chocolate candy

M & M's®, peanut	○		

Chocolate spread

Nutella®, chocolate hazelnut spread	○		

Dried fruit bars

Fruit Roll-Ups®			●

Nuts

Cashews	○		
Peanuts	○		
Pecans	○		

Popcorn

Plain, microwaved			●

Pretzels

Plain, salted			●

Snack bars

Apple Cinnamon, Con Agra	○		
Peanut Butter & Choc-Chip	○		
Twix® Cookie Bar, caramel	○		
Kudos Whole Grain Bars, chocolate chip		◑	

Sports bars

Ironman PR bar®, chocolate	○		

FOOD	LOW	INTERMEDIATE	HIGH
PowerBar®, chocolate		◐	

SOUPS

FOOD	LOW	INTERMEDIATE	HIGH
Lentil, canned	○		
Minestrone, canned, ready-to-serve	○		
Tomato, canned	○		
Black bean, canned		◐	
Green pea, canned		◐	
Split pea, canned		◐	

SPECIAL DIETARY PRODUCTS

FOOD	LOW	INTERMEDIATE	HIGH
Choice DM™, vanilla, Mead Johnson	○		
Ensure™, Abbott	○		
Ensure Plus™, vanilla, Abbott	○		
Ensure Pudding™, vanilla, Abbott	○		
Ensure™ bar, chocolate fudge brownie, Abbott	○		
Ensure™, vanilla, Abbott	○		
Glucerna™ bar, lemon crunch, Abbott	○		
Glucerna™ SR shake, vanilla, Abbott	○		
Glucerna™, vanilla, Abbott	○		
Resource Diabetic™, vanilla, Novartis	○		
Resource Plus, chocolate, Novartis	○		
Ultracal™ with fiber, Mead Johnson	○		
Enercal Plus™, Wyeth-Ayerst		◐	
Enrich Plus shake, vanilla, Ross		◐	

SUGARS

FOOD	LOW	INTERMEDIATE	HIGH
Blue Agave, Organic Agave Cactus Nectar, light, 90% fructose, Western Commerce	○		
Blue Agave, Organic Agave Cactus Nectar, light, 97% fructose, Western Commerce	○		

FOOD	LOW	INTERMEDIATE	HIGH
Fructose	◯		
Lactose	◯		
Honey		◑	
Sucrose		◑	
Glucose			●
Maltose			●

VEGETABLES

FOOD	LOW	INTERMEDIATE	HIGH
Artichokes	◯		
Avocado	◯		
Bok choy	◯		
Broccoli	◯		
Cabbage	◯		
Carrots, peeled, cooked	◯		
Cassava (yuca), cooked with salt	◯		
Cauliflower	◯		
Celery	◯		
Corn, canned, no salt added	◯		
Cucumber	◯		
French beans (runner beans)	◯		
Leafy greens	◯		
Lettuce	◯		
Peas, frozen, cooked	◯		
Pepper	◯		
Potato, sweet	◯		
Squash	◯		
Yam	◯		
Beet		◑	
Corn, sweet, cooked		◑	
Potato, boiled/canned		◑	
Potato, new, canned		◑	

FOOD	LOW	INTERMEDIATE	HIGH
Taro		◐	
Broad beans			●
Parsnips			●
Potato, French fries, frozen and reheated			●
Potato, instant			●
Potato, mashed			●
Potato, microwaved			●
Potato, Russet, baked			●
Pumpkin			●
Rutabaga			●

FOR MORE INFORMATION

To find a dietitian:
The American Dietetic Association
120 S. Riverside Plaza
Suite 2000
Chicago, IL 60606
Phone: 1-800-877-1600
www.eatright.org

**To order Natural Ovens bread
(available through mail-order only):**
Natural Ovens Bakery
PO Box 730
Manitowoc, WI 54221-0730
Phone: 1-800-772-0730
www.naturalovens.com

**To order Fifty50 Foods or find your
nearest retailer:**

Fifty50 Foods
PO Box 89
Mendham, NJ 07945
Phone: 1-973-543-7006
www.fifty50.com

ABOUT THE AUTHORS

JENNIE BRAND-MILLER, PH.D., is Professor of Human Nutrition in the Human Nutrition Unit, School of Molecular and Microbial Biosciences at the University of Sydney, and President of the Nutrition Society of Australia. She has taught postgraduate students of nutrition and dietetics at the University of Sydney for over twenty-four years and currently leads a team of twelve research scientists, whose interests focus on all aspects of carbohydrates—diet and diabetes, the glycemic index of foods, insulin resistance, lactose intolerance, and oligosaccharides in infant nutrition. She has published sixteen books and 140 journal articles, and is the co-author of all books in the *Glucose Revolution* series.

JOHANNA BURANI, M.S., R.D., C.D.E., is a Registered Dietitian and Certified Diabetes Educator with more than thirteen years of experience in nutritional counseling. The co-author of *The Glucose Revolution Life Plan* and *Good Carbs, Bad Carbs,* as well as several other books and professional manuals, she specializes in designing individual meal plans based on low-GI food choices. She lives in Mendham, New Jersey.

KAYE FOSTER-POWELL, M. NUTR. & DIET., is an accredited practicing dietitian with extensive experience in diabetes management. She has conducted research into the glycemic index and its practical applications over the last fifteen years. Currently she is a dietitian with Wentworth Area Diabetes Services in New South Wales and consults on all aspects of the glycemic index. She is the co-author of all books in the *Glucose Revolution* series.

SUSANNA HOLT, PH.D., works closely with Dr. Jennie Brand-Miller as the Research Manager of Sydney University's Glycemic Index Research Service (SUGiRS). She is also a qualified dietitian and nutrition consultant.

ACKNOWLEDGMENTS

WE WOULD LIKE to thank Linda Rao, M.ED., for her editorial work on the American edition.

Also Available

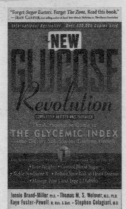

THE NEW GLUCOSE REVOLUTION

The Authoritative Guide to the Glycemic Index—the Dietary Solution for Lifelong Health

Written by the world's leading authorities on the subject, whose findings are supported by hundreds of studies from Harvard University's School of Public Health and other leading research centers, *The New Glucose Revolution* shows how and why eating low-GI foods has major health benefits for everybody seeking to establish a way of eating for lifelong health.

ISBN 1-56924-506-1 • $15.95

New York Times bestseller

THE GLUCOSE REVOLUTION LIFE PLAN

Discover how to make the glycemic index —the most significant dietary finding of the last 25 years— the foundation for a lifetime of healthy eating

More than

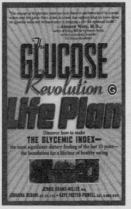

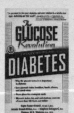
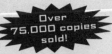
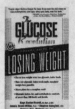
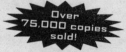

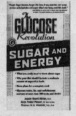

GOOD CARBS, BAD CARBS

▶ An accessible guide to help you
choose the right carbs.
ISBN 1-56924-537-1 • $9.95

Food manufacturers are showing increasing interest in having the GI values of their products measured. Some are already including the GI value of foods on food labels. As more and more research highlights the benefits of low-GI foods, consumers and dietitians are writing and telephoning food companies and diabetes organizations asking for GI data. This symbol has been registered in several countries, including the United States and Australia, to indicate that a food has been properly GI tested—in real people, not in a test tube—and also makes a positive contribution to nutrition. You can find out more about the program at www.gisymbol.com.au.

As consumers, you have a right to information about the nutrients and physiological effects of foods. You have a right to know the GI value of a food and to know it has been tested using appropriate standardized methodology.